PRESCRIPTION FOR A SUCCESSFUL CAREER IN MEDICINE

Essentials of the Health Care Profession

Jean Daniel François, M.D.

Printed in the United States of America
Revised Edition
Cover concept and design: Denise Gibson
ISBN: 978-09823142-2-7

Also by Dr. Jean Daniel François:

Prescription For A Successful Life

Les Clés de la Réussite Authentique

Prescription for an Exciting Love Life

You may visit the author's website,
www.successfullife.us or email him at
drfrancoismd@gmail.com

For information, to order additional books, or
for any other reasons, please write:
Jean Daniel François, M.D.
P.O. Box 360543
Brooklyn NY 11236
USA
718-531-6100

*This book is dedicated to my son
Jean Daniel François II, my
daughter, Sarah Jocelyne François,
Lorraine Alexis, and to others—
from the younger generation—who have
inspired me to write it.*

PRESCRIPTION FOR A SUCCESSFUL CAREER IN MEDICINE

Essentials of the Health Care Profession

Jean Daniel François, M.D.

Foreword

Although this book aims to guide high school and college students, graduates and others who are considering medicine as a career, it also raises issues that concern career driven people as a whole. We live in a challenging world. Knowledge in general, especially in the health field, is paramount for a well balanced life. In response to the various needs of different generations, here is a revised publication with more elaborated chapters to promote better decisions. For example, everyone should read the first chapter.

The primary goal of this revised edition of *Tips for a Successful Career in Medicine* is to make easily available much desired information gathered from different sources in order to help everyone find the right path; either as they are about to choose a profession in general, or a career change toward the health profession. In the United States, the health professional schools want candidates to focus on obtaining a baccalaureate degree that includes completing the required courses for their major and the prerequisite courses for their expected programs. Following, the candidates can pursue their choice to become either doctors of medicine, or osteopathic medicine (MD or DO), dental medicine (DDS and DMD), podiatric medicine (DPM), optometric medicine (OD) or veterinary medicine (DVM).

As always, many thanks to all of you who help me realize this product. Everything that is written is given only as advice. People should take it as such. Best of luck!

Acknowledgments

No words are strong enough to express my gratitude and my appreciation to Miss Lorraine Alexis for valuable suggestions and practical advice and Ms. Denise Gibson for her patience and professionalism.

I am also very grateful to Jean Daniel François II, my son—my first reader. I love to look at the awe on your face while talking to me. I hope I never disappoint you. You always challenge me to do and be the best. I am equally grateful to my daughter, Sarah Jocelyne François. I wish I had your gifted imagination, your magic way with words, and your great intelligence.

Disclaimer

This book is written to inspire young people to take a serious look at the opportunities available in medicine, when they face the delicate and difficult task of choosing a career. It is also a refresher lecture for those who are already engaged in the field. It can help many to avoid costly mistakes. The author does not claim any special influence on or privileged association with the institutions involved in selecting the candidates who are accepted to their schools. This book does not contain all the necessary information required for the medical subject.

Everyone should read all the pertinent gathered facts available to help them make the right choices according to their dreams, wishes, and preparation. Everyone should see to it that they are using the most current data to suit their needs. Nevertheless, this is a valuable tool—among others—in helping those who are considering medicine as a career as well as those who are already involved in such a profession and who may need further encouragement and guidance along the way.

Whatever level you have attained in the health care profession, or if you are just curious about it, reading this book should provide valuable insight, benefits, and encouragement.

Should you discover any mistakes, please do not hesitate to let us know. While every care has been taken to ensure accuracy, the author shall not be held responsible or liable to any person or institution regarding any loss or harm caused or alleged to have been due directly or indirectly to the information provided in this book.

Contents

"To find a career to which you are adapted by nature, and then to work hard at it, is about as near to a formula for success and happiness as the world provides. One of the fortunate aspects of this formula is that, granted the right career has been found, the hard work takes care of itself. Then hard work is not hard work at all."

~ Mark Sullivan

"Man is capable of doing countless things. Because of time confinement, he needs to pick what he is best at. The challenge is in finding it"

~ JDF

Prologue

Hi! Guess what? Good news!

You can be a Doctor! Yes, you can enjoy a great rewarding career in Medicine and love it! I know!

My mother always reminds me that I was six years old when I told her I wanted to be a doctor. But it took me three decades before I finally did it. Why? Here are a few reasons: fear of failing; ignorance; listening to so called friends, parents, advisors who were supposed to know more than I did; desire to please others; settling for the rat race; conformity; doubts; letting other people define me while they claim to know me more than I know myself—and a long list of other excuses. I am grateful to have come to my senses finally and to have followed my dream. I am happy to report to you that I do not regret yielding to my inner call. I am glad I still had that fire burning in me to leave other confused pathways and engage in medicine.

Perhaps you too are agonizing about the same dream. This is why I wrote this book—to provide at least a flickering light to help you get to the main road. It is written in the Holy Book: "my people are dying for lack of knowledge". For all the years I have been in medicine, I am always amazed to see so many young people including minorities who have a lot of potential but do not dare to consider getting involved in medicine, because of so much misconception. They do not know what to do or where to start. Unfortunately, even some of the advisors tend to guide the naïve students toward any made up major *ad libidum*. Sometimes, those who are there to help—for many reasons—misguide those poor young souls.

I still remember when I asked one chairman for a letter of recommendation to go to medical school. He told me through his glasses, "Come on! Get real, Jean. Why don't you do something else?" I do not believe this is an isolated incident. Some bright young students told me they had to keep their dream inside and could not even dare to express it until they met all the requirements. The time has come for people to know the truth about a career in medicine. It is a field available for all of those who hear the call and feel the urge to care for others.

Of course this book is by no means a comprehensive step-by-step guide to medicine. However, it is a stepping-stone in the right direction. I want to demystify the concept of admission to medical school for all who are considering such a call. I hope this book can lead the readers to resources available to help them make the right decision. They can also consult WWW.ASPIRINGDOCS.ORG and WWW.AAMC.ORG/STUDENTS.

By the way, let me point out again that this book is neither endorsed by nor has any affiliation with any medical school. I just feel compelled to make it available for those who want to take their first baby step towards medicine, who were afraid, overwhelmed by myths and unverified anecdotes. Let the journey begin!

Part 1:

Secrets To Get Into Medical School

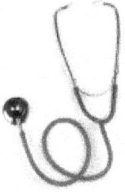

1
How to Choose a Career

It is eleven o'clock in the morning; Grandpa sits in his armchair, waiting to be picked up to go to the doctor. As often, Johnny jumps up and lands on his lap. He asks Johnny, "What do you want to do when you grow up?"

The face sparkling with delight and without hesitation, Johnny answers, "I want to be a doctor, to take care of you, Grandpa." They both laugh.

Grandpa says, "The other day you told me you wanted to be a fireman, then a policeman, then my barber, now a doctor, how many things do you plan to do, Johnny?"

The six-and-a-half-year-old answers, "I want to be all of those!"

All of us can remember how, as a child growing up, we wanted to be almost anything under the sun: Superman, fireman, doctor, lawyer, sportsman, or any of the popular stars seen on TV. To top it all off, every now and then we would meet people who would ask us who we want to become when we grow up. And depending on our mood and our state of mind, we would blurt out something that would either shock them or make them proud. Often, the adults would try, directly or indirectly, consciously or subconsciously, to influence us as to what our profession was going to be. Before we know it, those days are gone. We wake up one day and we discover we are young adults, middle aged or even counting the later years of our existence. All of us start with big dreams; all of us want to function within our expanded physical, financial, intellectual, emotional and cultural comfort zone. The truth of the matter is, time flies, unexpected, uninvited events do come in at any rate and gravity. We need to be well prepared. Our character, motivation, discipline, tenacity, ethic, education, experience, wisdom, maturity, decision, and attitude can lead us to make the key choices that will determine our destiny. The unprecedented advances in various areas of science, technology and education offer us different options in the selection of our profession. Nevertheless, the choice of a career remains a challenging and daunting task not to be taken lightly. This is usually a commitment for life. No one wants to repeat such an agonizing experience over and over again. Wouldn't it be great to make one choice, once in a lifetime, enjoy it, and stay with it until the end? Can we pick a career that provides a desirable standard of living in terms of place to live, family life, climate control, entertainment, health, and socioeconomic status...?

HERE ARE SEVEN BASIC PRINCIPLES THAT SHOULD GUIDE ANYONE IN THE CHOICE OF A CAREER:

1. *Identify yourself.* Know who you are. This is based on your genetic composition and vulnerability, family, environment, cultural and economic background, your personality and character, your age, creed, qualifications, competency, self-esteem, self-worth, self-actualization, and self-confidence. Also, how do others view you? What have you heard about your strengths and weaknesses? What environment fits you best? Be true to yourself; ask friends and families for their sincere input, but do not let anyone pressure you into choosing a profession. Remember, people can be biased or even jealous. It is your call and yours only. So be perfectly honest with yourself.

2. *Identify what you want in life.* What is it that, deep inside, you always long to do? What do you enjoy? What would you have fun doing even if

you had to spend your entire life doing it without any remuneration, under dire circumstances? If you were given the distinguished honor to make a significant change in this world, what would you want it to be and in what area?

3. *Be practical.* The marriage between what you want and what is applicable is not always an easy one. Take your time. Look around you and have a good grip on reality. This will give you an idea of what you like, as well as what is available that can make you useful in your environment and can positively impact your expected lifestyle and way of life.

4. *Discover what is required.* See what you need to do to be among the best in whatever it is that you choose to do. What are you lacking to fulfill your cherished dream? Take the necessary steps to be knowledgeable, qualified and well educated in whatever you choose to do. Always shoot for excellence!

5. *Identify resources.* Find out where you can get what you need to make your dream a reality and take the appropriate steps to get it without stepping on others' toes. You need to be weary about who is guiding you. Many times those who are engaged in counseling act and provide advice according to what they can see: your grades, your age, your economic or ethnic background. They may want to lead you towards what seems more practical but not necessarily what coincides with your deeply rooted dreams. There are instances when people who mean well may not be in tune with what you want. Make sure you take everything into consideration before you make your final decision.

6. *Identify the investment.* Because life is relatively short, one does not have a luxury to make too many mistakes and to have to start over. So, determine— as early and as thoroughly as possible—how much time, money, and energy you have accessible and

are willing to invest to get to where you want to be. Where would you get the needed support? Remember, any career you want to embrace, requires you to give it "your all" in order to be the best in it.

7. *Identify the rewards.* Identify the advantages and the disadvantages of your chosen profession for you and your significant others as well as the prospects for advancement. When you select one field, you let go of the opportunity to try another field. So be careful. Do not let money and glamour be your primary or sole motivations.

After doing all of the above and even more, take your time literally to investigate about each possible career, learn the pros and cons. Go through a process of elimination to bring the list down to 25, 20 and 10. Now from the 10 professions, try to narrow it down further. One approach is to adopt the familiar "one to ten scale". Then choose your most favorites and rate them as one, two, etc.

Ask yourself how much you want to do number one under any circumstances, why, for how long. Where do you see yourself in 5, 15, 25 years from now with that choice, while taking into consideration the life style, the place to live, family and relation situation, financial options, intellectual challenges...that you dream of. It may not be as easy as one may think when you have a choice. Many people find themselves in a situation where they were dropped into a job, or caged in. You do not want to do that. So, if you have the opportunity, make good use of it. Reading this book is a step in the right direction; but do not stop here. Do not leave any stone unturned until you find what you are really searching for. May your choice be according to your abilities, your cherished dreams, and with the proper unbiased guidance! I wish you the best of luck!

NOTES

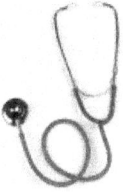

2

Reasons to Seek a Medical Career

What Makes You Decide To Go To Medical School?

The reasons are diverse and vary by individual. Some may want to save lives; others may hope to help the underserved or to compensate for the lack of care received by a love one; some may look forward to the knowledge, the privileges, or the responsibilities; some may want to further the research of a particular field; some may be following in the footsteps of a parent who is a healthcare professional.

No matter what, it is prudent to assume you have done your homework and now you are ready to embark in the most exciting journey of your life. The years in medical school will definitely change the way you think and the way you see others and yourself. But through it all you will always be dealing with people. You may have some doubts, so here are ten reasons why you should embrace medicine.

TEN REASONS WHY YOU SHOULD CONSIDER BECOMING A DOCTOR OF MEDICINE

1. The possibility to have a positive and meaningful impact in this world, to join a worthy and noble cause: if you are interested in making a difference in people's lives, it is an exciting and a challenging opportunity to make a meaningful contribution.

2. The possibility to be in a dynamic field with various specializations, promising prospects, and unlimited boundaries for unprecedented scientific progress and discoveries.

3. The possibility of stability and security to pursue the career at different levels and in different aspects of medicine—as an academician, scientist, researcher, writer, or clinician—or to obtain a combined MD/PhD, MD/JD, MD/MBA or MD/MPH, for example.

4. The ability to set your own objectives and to progress accordingly, either self-employed with your own practice or working for an established institution or both.

5. The possibility to find a specialization you like or a form of practice that feeds your type of personality and your needs, and be proactive.

6. The possibility—in many aspects—to choose where and what to practice and be a leader in your field.

7. The possibility to have financial stability, along with a decent lifestyle, as well as the privileges that go along with responsibilities.

8. The possibility for a lifelong learning experience: to increase your knowledge and improve your techniques; and to identify new approaches for the diagnosis and treatment of patients.

9. The possibility to enjoy a flexible schedule to adjust your lifestyle and balance academic pursuits with all the other things you love to do.

10. The possibility for personal gratification from providing outstanding services, networking and interacting with various specialties and scholastic colleagues.

MINORITY STUDENTS AND MEDICAL SCHOOL

If it is true that many young people are misinformed about their opportunities to go to medical schools and pursue their lifetime dream, minority students are no exception. As a matter of fact, a lot of them tend to shy away from medicine as if it were an unreachable dream. Nothing is further from the truth. The Association of American Medical Colleges in general, as well as most individual medical schools, are constantly and actively seeking to attract qualified minority students to the medical schools. Since the creation of AAMC Office of Minority Affairs in 1969, it has made it a prime objective—through reviewing government policies, assisting schools, informing potential candidates, and providing appropriate support—to spread the word, attract, accept, maintain, and graduate people from various under represented minority groups in the field of medicine. Through various publications, services, programs, workshops, counseling, college advisors, and college campus visits, information is made available to all who are interested in the medical field. There is a concerted effort by the AAMC and the individual colleges to attract, enroll, and train minorities from all groups including African Americans, American Indians, Hispanics, and women to find a career in medicine. Unfortunately, the individuals who are in an influential position for educating, advising, and guiding the minorities students do not always convey the proper encouragement; a few may not even be knowledgeable enough to provide much needed information to the right group of people who can really benefit from it. Some may have been discouraged by the disconnect between minorities in the health care profession in relation to minorities. Regardless of the causes, it is time for minorities to be exposed to the idea of embracing medicine on a regular basis instead of being directed towards other majors. They need mentors and inspirational role models in the field. Special thanks to those who have done it!

I sincerely hope there will be a direct and proportional trend between the percentage of minorities that make up the general population and the percentage of them who are encouraged to embrace medicine as their lifelong career. Overall, I strongly urge everyone in the new generation to consider seriously the health care profession as a definite and rewarding career.

NOTES

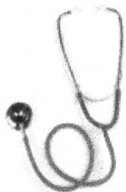

3
When Should You Prepare for Medical School?

The simple answer is as soon as possible. Once you are mature enough to think seriously about your career, you should explore all the possibilities. If you are geared towards medicine, then you should start gathering data, asking questions, visiting places, and trying to learn as much as possible about that field (but don't spend so much time on it that it has a negative effect on your overall performance in school). The sooner the better—in middle school, junior high, or high school, you should start to take steps in the right direction.

WHY DO PEOPLE USUALLY GO TO COLLEGE?

Most people say they go to college to further their education, get an under-graduate degree and be better qualified for a decent job. But many eighteen-year-old students may not even know why they are there. They want to get used to the new environment, adjust, skim the reading assignments, barely meet the deadline for homework, sleep late, get up just in time to make it to class before the "teacher with no life" marks them absent and penalizes them on the final grade, then party and enjoy life. It takes a while to realize the importance of what is being taught and take things a bit more seriously. The fact remains college is there to teach you how to think, read, write, and express yourself properly, behave like a mature person, and stay healthy and balanced physically and mentally, focusing on becoming a responsible citizen.

How To Be Ahead Of The Game

When you are privileged, somehow, to engage in a purposeful pathway, as a freshman with enough insight to work toward a career in medicine, you should inquire about the proper channel, secure a qualified advisor, and become familiar with certain websites, including www. aamc.org/students. You should consult the Association of American Medical Colleges current publications, the Annual Medical School Admission Requirements (MSAR), and other similar venues where you can find the lists of all the accredited United States medical schools. You should start choosing your outside activities, your volunteering, your community service, and your reading with an eye toward the medical field. As the semesters go by, you should try to complete the required premedical courses and degree requirements and to gather all the appropriate information. You should continue in such activities and plan to take the Medical College Admission Test (MCAT) in the spring of the third year or later that summer. You should remain in contact with your advisor for proper guidance to keep up to date, submit all the necessary documents on time, meet all the requirements, and get ready for the big leap in your life.

Speaking of getting ready, you should not ignore the financial aspect. The road to medical school is costly. You need to be prepared to spend money for MCAT, applications, prep courses, and prep books; add to this, secondary applications and traveling for interviews; these preliminary steps alone can cost you easily a couple of thousand dollars, or even more. So plan ahead and you won't have to let money stand in the way of pursuing your dream.

Methodically following these steps will make your preparation for a medical career a regular pathway and decrease the level of stress associated with it.

Notes

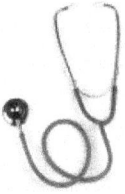

4

How to Position Yourself for Admission

So, you want to be a doctor of medicine! Congratulations! You have made a wise decision. Now, how do you get there?

SEVEN MYTHS ABOUT MEDICAL SCHOOL YOU NEED TO DEBUNK?

Myth #1 Only people who are extremely bright get admitted to medical school.

Truth: It is great to be very intelligent and to have excellent grades. But this is not a *sine qua non* for admission. Many people with average grades do get into medical school, because most institutions take into account a variety of factors for admission. Each candidate is considered for the various accomplishments and the circumstances in his or her life.

Myth #2 One must have money or be from a wealthy family to afford it.

Truth: Of course money does not hurt. But provisions are made to find ways to allow dedicated aspiring physicians to respond to their call, through loans and scholarships. This is where grades play a pivotal role because academic performance weight heavily for those who may otherwise be qualified, and are competing for scarce scholarships.

Myth #3 One must have a degree in science to make it.

Truth: Some credits are required in chemistry, biochemistry, biology, math, and physics. However it is not mandatory to have a major in science *per se* to be admitted to medical school. As a matter of fact, some schools are very much interested in other majors for some diversity in the classrooms, providing you are competent to handle the courses in medical school. Bear in mind, the common goal of the medical schools is to find candidates who are best suited not only to withstand the challenges during the four years in medical school, but who can respond to the ever growing needs of the society through their cognitive and acquired skills.

Myth #4 Admission is based on GPA and MCAT.

Truth: Again, it is great to have excellent grades and high MCAT scores. A decent minimum is required by most schools, because these grades tend to function as a way to anticipate the ability to handle the classes. But they are not the sole predictors for admission or rejection. Your record in the areas of clinical exposure, volunteering, research, shadowing, etc. will also have their role to play in the decision of the admissions committee.

*Myth #5 All medical schools are
         the same.*

Truth: Yes and no. Yes in a sense that
       once you are admitted to an
       accredited medical school in
       the United States and meet
       all the requirements, you are
       likely to go through the system,
       obtain your degree, get into
       a residency program and be
       rewarded a license to practice
       medicine. No, because there are
       some differences in what specific
       schools put more emphasis on.
       For example, some schools
       are more clinically oriented
       others more academically oriented
       or more research oriented. So,
       if ever you have a choice, you
       should pick the one that fosters
       mostly what you are interested in,
       that has a great reputation with
       an ideal location for you and at
       the least cost possible.

*Myth #6 One must graduate from an
         Ivy League medical school to be
         a great physician.*

Truth: All medical schools that are
allowed to function officially in
the United States of America
are accredited, whether or not
they are in the Ivy League.
Because every year many highly
qualified students are not selected,
wherever you are accepted in the
system, be glad to attend and do
your utmost to learn as much as
possible, to find your niche, to excel
in what you are most compelled
to do, and to become a competent
physician. If given a choice,
obviously it is worth going for a
top rated, prestigious institution.

Myth #7 *It takes too many years of
studying; one must be fresh out
of college, in their early twenties
to be a serious contender.*

Truth: What we do with our time
is essential in our existence.
However, if we do nothing,
time will still pass us by.
Unfortunately, many people
choose to spend time recklessly.
Going to medical school is an

investment for a rewarding, exciting, and honorable passage. The time spent in medical school contributes to your intellectual, mental, social, and cultural upbringing. After four years in medical school, you get paid to learn as a resident. How many professions can do this for you? Of course, age plays a role in learning and performance. But it can also work in your favor. Each case is evaluated and studied individually. If you are in your thirties for example, it would be interesting to find out what you have been doing with your life. If the answer is credible, genuine, and acceptable, you will definitely find medical schools that are interested in you.

Please do not forget that some U.S. institutions give the option to begin medical school right after high school. This allows you to get an MD degree in 6 to 8 years after high school.

The rules for admission to medical schools are not set in stone. A few factors that are taken into consideration. They usually want to see the whole picture and determine whether or not you will be able to obtain the grades and stay in school once you are selected; and go on to become a dignified servant of the community through your knowledge, skills and manners.

WHAT ARE THE STEPS TO BE ADMITTED INTO MEDICAL SCHOOL?

By the time you decide to choose a career in the medical field, you are likely to be in college. But ideally you should begin earlier. This will make you more careful in class attendances, the management of your courses, withdrawals, incomplete and unsatisfactory performance, the choice of your electives, where to invest your leisure time, and the type of activities you should be involved in; and you will pay closer attention to your grades. At any rate, no one is perfect, the past is gone. Now is the moment to make the most of what is available to you. It is the time to reflect on your past, your previous accomplishments.

To have reached that crossroad, you need to be proud of yourself. The best years of your life are ahead of you, filled with excitement, knowledge, and challenges. So get ready to cross the bridge safely, with enthusiasm and determination. It is worth pointing out that Medicine is a life time career. After high school, you begin with 4 years of college, 4 years in medical school, then a minimum of 3 years of residency that can extend between 4 and 6, based on the specialty you are interested in. If you know early enough about your choice for medicine, you may apply to some US medical schools that accept people in their program right after high school with the ability to receive their MD diploma after 6 to 8 years. Furthermore, after graduation, your options include private practice (solo or group), academic pursuits, teaching, research, or working for institutions such as hospitals, HMO, government or military, or even a mixed bag that suits your needs and desires.

Except for a few changes, most medical schools have a set of criteria for admissions.

1. You must complete science courses with lab work to meet the premedical curriculum requirements. The courses include one year each, with lab performance where appropriate, in general biology, physics, inorganic chemistry, organic chemistry, and English. In addition, courses in behavioral sciences, other health-science related subjects, and humanities; including languages, writings. Maths...also play their role.

2. You must have a bachelor of arts or bachelor of sciences degree.

3. You must take the Medical College Admission Test before the applications deadline, usually within the previous three years (a few places do not require the MCAT exam prior to the application).

4. For the sake of completeness, allow me to point out that you should always aim at applying when you feel you are best prepared. Although the convention is to get things ready by the end of your junior year, you should

not be pressured to take the MCAT when you are not well prepared and would have to take it again. You may need to finish with classes that you believe will increase your chances of improving your scores in sciences, writing or verbal reasoning, or even making a better impression to the medical schools you want to apply to.

5. Obviously, you must be a United States citizen or a legal resident. The competition is very tight and the expenses are high even for these candidates.

6. You must have at least three letters of recommendations from the best qualified professors, preferably those on your advisory committee, including the chairman in a science department. Show good judgment by choosing not only those who can write excellent letters but those with respectable positions in the school and the department where you majored. One of the ways to obtain such letters is to be able to have those professors remember your name and face.

In huge classes, the key is to take time to go to the office after hours and show that you are interested in the subject without making any waves, or bragging about your intelligence.

Be organized! See to it that all transcripts, letters, and supporting documents are submitted in a timely fashion. Make a list of the schools you want to apply to; then fill out and submit the appropriate applications on time, before the deadline, and check to see that they are received. Many schools will send out their own application also, to be filled out promptly, and may require a non-refundable application or processing fee.

To avoid any mishap, you must keep a list of all the required documents together with proof of timely submission for each. Remember, the schools have not met you yet. But what you submit, when and how you submit it already gives them an idea as to whether or not you will fit into the student body they are trying to attract and prepare for medicine.

After you have taken all the steps and submitted all documents, you have to get ready for the interviews. Do not call the schools to remind them. Do not irritate any personnel by nagging them or complaining to them for not calling you early enough. This would definitely give them a negative vibration towards you as one of their students. Nevertheless, you may decide to send an 'update card' just to tell them about new credits, new accomplishments and kindly remind the school that you are still interested.

Early decision: If you fall in love with a campus and you are determined to be admitted there, you can submit your application for early decision. You should avoid being accepted in more than one school when it comes to early admission. Make sure that a given school processes your application early enough (ideally, within the first few weeks when application acceptance begins) so that you can still apply to the general pool of students as one of the regular candidates, if things do not work out as expected on either side.

Notes

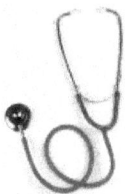

5

How to Be Among the Top Candidate for Any Medical School

Some people wonder why it is so hard to get accepted into medical school. As a matter of fact, for every candidate accepted, two are likely to be rejected. The answer is based on a simple old economic principle: the law of supply and demand. On the one hand, there are a lot of very bright college students who "demand" entry; on the other hand, there is a limited "supply" of medical schools available to accept them. So, every year, medical schools throughout the United States of America and also in Canada; have the herculean task of selecting a limited number of students from among thousands of well-qualified candidates. How do they decide to accept one candidate and reject another one?

Here is a list of factors that determine such a choice:

1. **Educational background**. They look for a broad educational preparation that includes not only the required courses but also classes in other areas capable of making the candidate a well-rounded person whose intellectual capacities are wide and deep. Grades are important; you should do your best to keep your GPA above a 3. But, the schools also take into consideration the length of time spent to earn the degree, the number of credits taken per semester, classes from which the student had to withdraw, repeated courses, and the number of incomplete courses (this may reflect your discipline, your study habits, and your level of persistence and motivation and may give an idea of your overall academic ability to face the rigor of medical education).

2. **The College attended.** The grades obtained, including respectable MCAT scores, help the school to anticipate ability to perform well academically. Overall, straight A's in an average college may be better

appreciated in some institutions than a collection of C's and W's (withdrawals) in a well-respected, reputable college. It all depends on your overall achievement in life.

3. **Extracurricular activities.** The medical school is interested in what else you have done besides being a bright student. If you have spent your entire life as a bookworm, some may wonder how you can apprehend the various aspects of medicine and its numerous challenges. It is a big plus to be able to show that since high school— or even before—you were involved in some community activities such as: fighting illiteracy or child abuse, disease prevention, hunger prevention, volunteering in a nursing home or a medical office, assisting the elderly, or crisis intervention. Such activities are characteristic of a dedicated, altruistic person who is really interested in making a difference in people's lives.

4. **Life experience, maturity and responsibilities.** One of the key challenges of the admissions committee

is to pick those with the personal and emotional stability to stay the course during the four years in medical school, where people are undoubtedly going to be under a lot of pressure and have to accomplish a lot. So, the extent and length of your past experience, the types of responsibilities you have had, and their impact on your personal life would give an idea of the type of person you are and your leadership skills. Your unique life history, the trials and tribulations you have overcome, the tests of life you have endured steadfastly can put them at ease. Remember, most candidates have great GPAs and excellent MCAT scores, in some instances even better than you do. Your personal history, your personal touch, your ability to convey who you are in the best light possible without being pompous but with humility, your acquired skills in the health domain, your views and commitment *vis-à-vis* your community and the role of medicine make the difference. You must be able to exploit your apparently disadvantageous situation (if any) in order to brand it as a plus, a steppingstone toward reaching your goal.

5. **Diversity.** Discrimination because of your age, race, creed, sexual orientation, gender, religion, country of origin, or disability is legally prohibited. Bear in mind, we are dealing with human beings who naturally tend to be biased in one way or another. So be truthful but be moderate. If you happen to belong to a group that is underrepresented or underprivileged, do not let that stop you. As a matter of fact, many institutions aim at having a well balanced, diverse, and truly representative multicultural community as possible.

6. **Personal Statement.** As stated, your personal statement tells a school about what is unique not weird or peculiar about you. It should present you in the best favorable manner possible. So take your time to find the best way to convey the pertinent facts about you. Make it your blue print (if not your fingerprint). You

need to find a unique way to say a lot about you without writing too much. So it is not only what you say but how you manage to express it in order to make a reader want to know more about you, and want to give you an interview. This personal statement may be the bridge you walk on to get to the interview. If you need extra help, remember there are qualified organizations and people out there to help. Make sure you get the right and reasonable one.

7. **Meeting the requirements.** The timing of the submission of your documents, the quality of your documents, and your personal statements build that bridge on which you can walk to the interview. So beware of what you submit, what you write, how you write it, and how you present it. Be sincere, genuine, organized and straightforward. Explain clearly why you want to be a physician, why you want to attend their particular school, and why you want them to choose you as one of their students.

8. **The interview.** Although a few schools may interview every applicant who is a state resident, most of them will not go through all the steps and review all the records just to call you for chitchat. By the same token, although you have become a serious contender, you are not there yet. Hold on to the celebration. Be careful not to blow it. Remember the schools want to make sure they have the best students. They do not have a crystal ball to see the future. So they are relying on certain criteria, certain personality traits to cast their ballots for or against your application. The face-to-face interview is your unique opportunity to make the best impression on your interviewer or interviewers and seal your admission to that school. Of course you are both excited and nervous. You do not know what to expect, and so on and so forth. The bottom line: you get to be interviewed. So what do you do?

STEPS FOR THE INTERVIEW

1. **Prepare yourself mentally and physically.** When you are contacted for an interview, you need to remember this should be an exciting but a pleasant experience. The interviewers are not going to invite you to accuse or condemn you. So be relaxed. At this stage in your determination to get admitted into medical school, you should be prepared to tell anyone about yourself; why you want to be a doctor, what is unique about you, what specialty (if any) you are interested in and why, what makes a great doctor, your exposure to the medical field, what you would do if you do not get admitted (causing harm to yourself is not an option), your strengths, and how to point out your weakness and make it sound like a strength. For example: "I have a tendency, when I start something, not to take a break until I finish it"; "people tell me I am too disciplined"; "I keep a daily log of my activities and I am too conscious about the use of my time". But please

avoid giving an impression that you are just using a formula, a *cliché* to get by. Fidgeting, hesitating, playing with your pen, looking away, biting your nails, your body language, your voice...may convey a different message. Again, be genuine.

Be careful about how you approach controversial issues such as euthanasia, abortion, cloning, and so forth. But you should have an opinion about the current condition of the health care system.

Do you have a special person in your life who tends to influence you or inspire you? This is a common question that you may be asked, and you should think about an answer.

Review your application, your personal letter, and all the documents submitted to avoid contradicting yourself, leaving people wondering whether you have a clone or a split personality. Locate the place before the date of the interview, and sleep well (six to eight hours) the night before. Know a thing or two about the place you are going to. Make sure you are abreast of the current, relevant news, what is hot in the news about medicine, the new scientific discoveries, and so on. You are not expected to know every detail, but some basic information will impress your interviewer. You should be aware of some political issues, the position of a given candidate on stem cell research for example, how the local politicians view research, and other significant issues facing the scientific community. Most of this information is given regularly in the national and local news.

2. **Be aware of your appearance.** Dress appropriately—modestly and conservatively, meaning you should avoid showing off your body, avoid being too flashy, avoid wearing loud outfits. Dressing according to the season and age, what is fashionably acceptable and like other interviewees is a safe approach. Good personal hygiene is important, but avoid heavy perfume; take care of your hair, nails, and breath; the teeth and shoes should be clean. Have enough money; including some change for any unexpected

development such as metered or paid parking. No need to display all your electronic gadgets. Have your cell phone or beeper off. If possible, avoid an empty or a too full stomach; avoid taking new medicine for the first time because you do not know if it may affect your cognitive ability and your behavior. If the interview is out of town, avoid traveling the same day as much as possible.

3. **Show up on time**, or even a few minutes early, to find parking, to freshen up and fix yourself appropriately, to locate the floor, the department and the person whom you are going.

4. **Take a deep breath.** Drink some water, if available, and then walk steadily in a comfortable pair of shoes, with a winner's attitude. Be yourself and be ready to give it your best shot.

5. **Knock politely** and wait to be invited to enter, if applicable.

6. **Introduce yourself** to whomever you first meet, and give a firm

handshake (but do not break anyone's fingers), while smiling and looking the interviewer in the eye.

7. **Let the interviewer engage the conversation** and indicate to you where you should be seated. Do not move the chair any closer than where he or she puts you. Watch how you sit and how you project yourself.

8. **Sit comfortably** and remain calm, confident, pleasant and interesting.

Remember that during the first couple of seconds, interviewers measure you up to form a first impression. They are sizing you up. They want to check your demeanor, intelligence, communication skills, body language, emotions, listening skills, level of motivation, and ability to handle challenges and controversies. So be natural, and take your time to understand and answer each question. Remember you are not running for a political office. You must answer the basic questions. Some interviewers may even challenge you, in order to evaluate your thinking pattern and see how alert and sharp you are.

Expect to tell a few interesting things about yourself, some unique life experience that may lead you to be interested in the medical field, your plan for your life, the number of schools you have applied to, the interviews you have lined up or have had, what you like about their specific school, whether you would commit yourself to their school if accepted. The bottom line is that you must show your interest; be genuine, keep the answers short and straight to the point, and talk decisively and at a comfortable, audible level.

Ask a couple of intelligent questions regarding research, campus activities, scholarship and rewards for excellent performance, etc; even if you may have an idea about the answers.

There is no need to tell them every detail of your personal life, just whatever is relevant to give you an edge and get you closer to admission at their institution.

Do not criticize or put down any other institution, college, any part of the country, any religion, or any sexual orientation. Be neutral and talk passionately about your sense of purpose in life. By all means, do not be negative. Do not join the interviewer in complaining how bad things are, or that this is the end of the world. Be positive and enthusiastic. Don't run on beyond reason, but do not be too brief in your answers either. Speak with a light spirit and a naturally pleasant smile.

As much as it is possible, avoid scheduling two interviews in the same day. Do not keep checking your watch. Let the interviewer see you off, but do not take the initiative to say, for instance, "well, I guess that's set, I'll see you around, I have another interview in 5 minutes. Let me know if you want me. Bye!" You cannot do it that way.

Different interviewers may put you through different types of interviews. Some questions may test your common knowledge or your memory; others may check for your skills and competency. Let's say they ask you a question out of left field; you have no clue. What do you do? Do not panic. Try not to look unprepared; remain candid but upbeat. No matter what, never lose your self-confidence. If you really do not know the answer, be truthful, and use some clean humor when possible.

After the interview, the admissions committee will let you know about their decision. If it is in your favor, you have a few days or weeks to acknowledge the acceptance and confirm your intent to be part of that institution.

PERSONAL TESTIMONY

My passion for medicine goes as far back as I can remember in my childhood. My brothers and sisters used to tease me for the stupid things I used to say, I was willing to do anything to be sure I became a doctor. But growing up, listening to people, including my own father, I became confused, doubtful, overwhelmed. So I took accounting in college, switched to business, then got a master's in economics and worked in the business and accounting world just to make a living. Yet I was uncomfortable and literally lost. Something was missing. But by then I had already wasted quite a few years. To top it all, My GPA and my MCAT were not among the best. I was always working full time. Based on all the things I heard about medical school, I thought I was doomed. The only thing I had going for me was my leadership skills, my involvement in my community and my ability to perform several tasks at the same time including raising a family, going to school and working full time. This was not much at all.

Then some guy called me "doctor" by mistake at an event I attended. That was it! It clicked! I regained my self-confidence, my determination. I made the decision to get to medical school and pursue my childhood dream.

I had no coach, no mentor; as a matter of fact, I became a bit secretive about it because of all the negative feedback I got initially. I did not want to hear anything negative anymore. Except for my spouse, those who knew my plan thought I was crazy. But I was so fired up, nothing could stop me anymore. Based on my personal situation and obligations, I targeted three states and I applied to only ten schools. Once I was invited by two of them to be interviewed, I did not follow up with the rest (I should have).

When I went to the first interview, (in a neighboring state), it was snowing heavily. I showed up, but the interviewer did not. I had to reschedule. I was not impressed and did not follow through with that one either (I should have). So, practically, I had only one interview; and that one medical school accepted me. The rest is history.

Call it a miracle, faith, attitude, or anything else. I am happy to report to you, I am now living my dream. I am very grateful for that. Of course, everyone's situation is unique; but that was my personal journey with various detours.

So perseverance, discipline, confidence, and faith in yourself, your skills, talents, and faith in a higher power can make the difference.

Notes

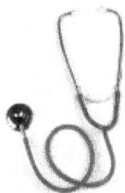

6
How to Stay in Medical School and Graduate

Finally, the long awaited envelope comes. What does it say? If it is negative, it is only saying "be back next year!" So you have another year to prepare yourself, get some more experience, and become more mature and better qualified. In all probability, if you follow the proper steps, if the time and circumstances are right, you are likely to be accepted by one medical school of your choice. The second time around may increase the odds in your favor. It reveals your character, your perseverance to get into the medical field.

Be it the first, the second or the third time, once you are admitted, it is a gigantic step in the right direction. You need to be prepared not only to be admitted to medical school but also to stay in school and to pass the courses until graduation four years later, when you attend the commencement of your medical journey, which will be full of excitement one way or the other. Your decision to go to medical school was not an easy one, but it was the right one. You have been realistic and practical; you know yourself and your personality; you are people-oriented and independent-minded; you like what is intellectually challenging and ambitious; you are dynamic and bright; and you choose to acquire enough knowledge to be better qualified to make a difference in alleviating human sufferings. This is commendable! Now you need to be intellectually and mentally prepared to stay up to the challenges.

Believe me, the first week in medical school will be an eye-opener. If you are not careful, the first few weeks or months may knock your socks off in amazement. But remember, you went through enough challenges to get there. So roll up your sleeves and get to it. If it helps you to know this, I must confess I thought I was the brightest kid in town until I went to medical school. When I failed my first test in histology, I wanted to quit.

I am grateful for all the support I received to help me proceed. I am glad I did.

Except for a few variations, most four-year medical schools make you spend the first two years studying basic science. This entails, for the first year: gross anatomy, histology and cell biology, biochemistry, physiology, neuroscience, and behavioral science. The second year consists of pharmacology, pathology and pathophysiology, microbiology and immunology, and physical diagnosis.

You need to pass your courses to advance to the next level. You also take your USMLE, step 1.

In the third and fourth year you are doing mostly clinical rotations in various hospitals that are available and associated with your medical school. You are really seeing the practical side of medicine by doing clinical rotation in internal medicine, obstetrics and gynecology, pediatrics, psychiatry, surgery, family medicine, and neurosurgery; and you venture into some electives to see what it is that you can choose to do eventually if you have not made up your mind already. But how do you stay in good standing in medical school for four years until you receive your diploma?

You have heard it before, nevertheless it is worth repeating: the four years in medical school are guaranteed to change your life, hopefully for the better. You are going to be amazed as to the quantities of information, knowledge, and skills acquired in so little time. How do you digest them and apply them? How do you grasp them so you can pass the tests to show how much you have been able to learn and to use appropriately? This is the most challenging phase of the medical student's life.

THE GOLDEN RULES TO SURVIVE MEDICAL SCHOOL

1. **Time management.** You will be bombarded by all kinds of information and requirements. You can be easily overwhelmed. You need to know early enough how to allocate your time: time to go through the materials from class and not let them pile up; time for class; time to study; time to sleep; and time to remain as a functional, decent, and sane human being.

2. **Revision of your ways of studying.** Network. Review and upgrade those

habits that used to work in the past. This is a brand new ball game. In medical school, you cannot do it alone. You must have a group of classmates— if not your lab group—then choose a few people you can get along with, preferably with different backgrounds and strengths in various subjects, so that you can help each other.

3. **Humility.** Be humble or set yourself up to be humiliated. First you will discover, maybe for the first time, that you can fail a course unless you seek appropriate help, no matter how bright your mother told you that you were. Second, professors, attending physicians, clerks, patients, and anybody around will tell you strange things or do humiliating things to you, and you won't be able to do much about it. But overall, it will be very exciting and rewarding, a great learning experience. If you are humble, respectful, and eager to learn, things will be easier for you. People will want to help you. No arguments, please!

4. **Responsibility.** Take your learning experience into your own hands. It is like erecting a building: you need a solid foundation. So take the two years of basic science very seriously. You will need them later on and may not have time to go back to them. Learn your anatomy, pathology, neuroscience, pharmacology, biology, biochemistry and all the rest. They are relevant for your formation.

5. **Learn what the scoop is to pass your classes.** Even though you know you are great, buy the transcripts of all the lectures that fellow classmates prepare from the lectures presented in class. If you are part of those who prepare them, do a good job, please! Buy the recommended textbook for the class. Get the general Board Review books. Resist the urge to buy every book under the sun for every subject. All in all, you need to know the materials and to explore the subjects; usually the recommended textbooks can help you in that domain. But you should find out for yourself the best way to handle each class.

6. **Be disciplined.** Identify what really works well for you. Use whatever is available that can make the difference for you. Attend lectures, labs, clinical case presentations, radiology conferences, and module presentations—anything that can make a positive difference in your student career—while maintaining a regular life as much as possible, keeping in touch with friends and family, and taking advantage of their much needed support.

7. **Get help if you need it.** Do not play hero. Do not rely on your friends' comments. They may be struggling like you, and you may not know it. Go to the appropriate departments' services, and they will be glad to help you swim through by advising you appropriately. Do not keep to yourself and sink or explode.

8. **Keep track of your financial status.** An increasing number of people who go to college wind up with a considerable amount of outstanding debt to be paid. Going to medical school is likely to

add on to your debt load. You know it already: education in general is expensive, medical school, even more. Many applicants are likely to be admitted to a private medical school. Generally, private schools are more expensive. This means a proportional increase in your loan and ultimately your debts. Do not damage your credit records. Pay all your bills on time. Avoid unnecessary debts.

You need to have a plan before you even start medical school. How are you going to pay for it? The bulk of your medical school education is likely to be financed by loans. But if your credit records are messed up, if you already owe a lot of money from your credit cards, this will make the situation even tougher. Remember, you are not likely to be able to work while going to classes, especially at the beginning.

There are nationwide financial aid programs, but they are limited. Bear in mind, not only do you have to pay for tuition; you also need books and must face living expenses and personal responsibilities. The medical schools have student financial assistance programs in which every condition is taken into consideration; and wherever appropriate, a need-based award scholarship is considered. Traditional and non-traditional financial aid resources in the form of grants and loans are available based on citizenship, state residency requirements, personal and parental financial status. There are some specific conditions attached to them, but you should be diligent enough to find ways to get through the medical school.

You should be aware of service agreements. As a matter of fact, there are some government aid projects and military service, where your tuition can be paid. There are some loan forgiveness programs, if you commit yourself to work in an underserved area for a specific number of years. This is another way to help you with the cost while helping the needy, the underprivileged people. Consult the Health Professions Scholarship Program (HPSP), AAMC website and other scholarship programs for further details. "Where there is a will, there is a way".

It is absolutely, positively important to be very careful as to the ways the loans and scholarship money are spent. Remember, all loans need to be repaid. So refrain from impulsive buying such as going for expensive cars, clothes, gifts, parties and gadgets. Please, even when the loan is available; use only the bare minimum that is absolutely necessary. Do not blow it quickly and have to struggle later to pay it back. Available money is like water on a dry land. You never know what happens to it, until the day of reckoning when you have to sweat and struggle to pay it back.

Have a budget and stick to it. Do not spend just to feel good; show off now and later you may explode. Resist the urge to be like your roommates, classmates, or friends. You do not know their financial conditions. Focus on yours and learn to live within your means, sometimes even below your means. Later on, looking back, you will be glad you did. But if you spend like there is no tomorrow, then you will have moments of sorrow. So, resist the spending impulse as much as possible.

Notes

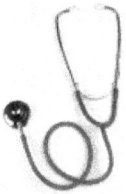

7
Why Not Be a Doctor of Osteopathic Medicine?

A significant number of people go to see their doctor without knowing whether or not the doctor who has been taking care of them is an MD or a DO. A recent study reveals that "doctor of osteopathic medicine" is not well grasped by the majority. People usually picture a doctor as someone with a white lab coat, who wears glasses, has a few grey hairs, a stethoscope around the neck, a penlight, and a lot of pens in their left breast pocket. What about you? What do you know about osteopaths? Have you seriously considered applying for a doctor of osteopathic medicine program? Why not? If you are dedicated, compassionate, and caring, with the aptitude and the desire to work in the health field with a lifelong commitment to health promotion and illness prevention; if you believe the human body's systems are interconnected with a whole person approach; if you are willing to learn how to use your ears, hands, and eyes to identify patients' conditions; if you see everyone as a whole, including nerves, muscles, bones, and organs, along with emotional and spiritual components; if you have or can develop a gentle touch and can learn the internal relationships between structure and function, you are the perfect candidate for osteopathic medicine. After all, as we navigate through life, we need to have dreams, but we also must have plans to make them a reality. Every year, a great number of excellent candidates cannot find a spot in the US or Canadian medical schools. If after you have done all that you could you are still waiting, perhaps it is because you do not know enough about alternatives. Osteopathic Medicine is a reasonable and even competitive alternative.

WHAT IS OSTEOPATHIC MEDICINE, ANYWAY?

In 1874, after some major disappointments with the results of traditional medicine, a medical doctor, Andrew Taylor Still, decided to reflect on the impact of medicine and to consider alternative ways to get better results in savings people's lives. He came up with a new approach in which, instead of focusing on isolated diseases, instead of considering each case as separated, Dr. Still wanted to put the emphasis on seeing the human being as a whole and to take steps toward re-establishing the harmony between body, mind, and spirit.

Instead of reacting when facing each situation, he wanted to take the necessary steps towards preventative medicine. This idea was familiar from the time of Hippocrates. In 1892, Dr. Still began the first college of osteopathy, in Kirksville, Missouri. Needless to say, at the beginning, he was a potential threat, and with the normal tendency for people to resist change, because of fears and politics, osteopathic medicine started as a struggle. The beginning was not easy and Dr. Still (an MD, you'll recall) had to fight off numerous attacks, including those legislative in nature. However, by the early 1970s, doctors of osteopathic medicine obtained full practice rights throughout the United States of America.

Nowadays, it is reported that there are well over 50,000 osteopathic physicians, graduates of twenty accredited osteopathic medical colleges, taking care of countless number of people throughout the United States. When it comes to competency and professionalism, no one can detect the difference.

You may be pleasantly surprised to know that, officially, there are two kinds of physicians equally qualified to practice medicine in all fifty states:

- **MD:** Doctor of allopathic medicine (treatment of disease by producing a condition incompatible with that disease)

- **DO:** Doctor of osteopathic medicine (aiming at keeping normal structural condition, normal body mechanics, using manipulative methods of detecting and correcting faulty structure)

Furthermore, MD and DO programs have a lot of similarities. Both require the following:

- **Completion of a bachelor's degree with successful completion of general biology, organic chemistry, general chemistry, and physics, with appropriate labs, along with classes in English.**

- **Taking the MCAT (scores not over three years old).**

- **Valuable letters of recommendation.**

- **Interview as part of the admission process.**

- **A competitive admission process.**

And the programs have additional similarities upon admission:

- **Both MD and DO programs last four years. The first two years are dedicated to basic science courses. During the third and fourth year the emphasis is on mandatory and elective clinical courses.**

- **Upon graduation, both DO and MD have the privilege of choosing their specialties for their residency.**

- **Both programs allow the candidates to submit and meet state and national requirements for licensing.**

- **Both can prescribe and perform the procedures that fall within their training.**

- **Both can work in any medical institutions and work side-by-side under one roof.**

- **Legally, both are equal and have the same responsibilities.**

If any difference must be noted, it may be to the advantage of the doctor of osteopathic medicine. They incorporate osteopathic manipulative treatment (OMT) in the training and practice of osteopathic physicians. They are prepared with the mindset of seeing patients as a whole, to be concerned about their entire body, mind, and soul, and with ways to help in prevention. While MDs see themselves as coaches to their patients, DOs consider themselves partners to their patients.

Nevertheless, as time goes by and the needs for complete care become more and more urgent, the differences tend to diminish. Nowadays, any experienced MD knows if a female patient comes in for headaches, the doctor needs to find out what is going on emotionally, her sleeping habits, history of trauma, cervical spine condition, nutritional status, food and eating habits, birth control pills, menstrual cycle, metabolic condition, and basic labs as a minimum. Otherwise, the physician writes prescription after prescription without any lasting results. Both of them (patient and doctor) will be frustrated. Today's doctors know about bedside manner and communication skills. On the other hand, the DOs tend to follow the trend of the MDs, with generally less manipulation than before, especially when manipulation performed is not billed as a separate procedure, while there is a slight risk of possible adverse effects to the point that only qualified doctors in the field of osteopathic medicine are allowed to perform manipulation. By the same token, DOs may have an edge with patients who love a personal touch and prefer doctors who lean towards natural medicine. Osteopathic medicine is enthusiastically acclaimed by a category of patients who show resistance to drugs or surgery. They see it as a welcome alternative. The DOs have two hundred to five hundred hours of extra training in the art of osteopathic manipulative medicine, mastering the musculoskeletal system to help them have a better understanding of the ways one affected part of the body can have its repercussion on the entire body. A lot of them specialize in the primary care areas of internal medicine, family practice, obstetrics and gynecology, and pediatrics. They are providing a much needed exemplary service to places of greatest need—small towns and the underserved and rural areas where they care for families and entire communities. But if they choose otherwise, they can pick any specialty and practice the full scope of modern medicine anywhere in the United States.

In this twenty-first century, the nation has to face the challenge of physician workforce shortage while keeping up with all the changes in modern medicine. The only two types of physicians licensed to practice medicine in all fifty states must play their part in providing outstanding care for all. If osteopathy was initially a drugless way to provide care, today's osteopathic physician's approach is not much different from the traditional MD's. They are complete physicians, highly qualified, and a rapidly growing force, accounting for nearly twenty percent of current medical students.

The trend is likely to remain upward. Osteopathic medicine, like allopathic medicine, wants to attract people with humanitarian and intellectual qualities, who want to remain at the cutting edge in academic excellence, provide outstanding clinical care, participate in ongoing research, commit to lifelong community service, and improve the health care system as a whole.

So if you are ready to consider each patient as a complete human being, if you care for a broad educational background, including a holistic view to diagnose and treat illness and injury, if you are ready to be part of a team of dedicated, passionate, and disciplined professionals, then becoming a doctor of osteopathic medicine is a viable alternative.

If you still have any doubt, then take the following steps: volunteer in a health care center where you can shadow a DO in action, get some information about the osteopathic medical profession (American Osteopathic Association), learn and evaluate the different osteopathic medical schools in the United States, learn about the four-years studies, and compare them with the regular medical schools. Weigh the benefits and limitations in the field, find out about tuition and fees and financial aid packages, get in touch with the American Association of Colleges of Osteopathic Medicine Application Service (AACOMAS, 301-968-4190, or WWW.AACOM.ORG), and talk to your family and friends after revealing the true facts about doctors in osteopathic medicine. Osteopathy is here to stay and to flourish.

The practice of osteopathic medicine in the United States generally includes the same techniques, prescriptions, and risks as that of medical doctors. DOs and MDs may belong to two different branches of the American medical care system, but they work together to provide the much needed care nationwide.

All in all, if Dr. Still, MD, the pioneer in osteopathic medicine was ostracized in the late 1800s, if some may still have objections and mostly unfounded criticism, if others need time to grasp the concept, if it still meets some resistance and may face some prejudice, the fact is the doctor in osteopathic medicine is qualified and recognized in all fifty states with the same rights, privileges, and responsibilities as the medical doctor. They too are committed to serving the health care needs of the nation. Therefore, anyone who is interested to work in the medical field has the opportunity to consider becoming either MD or DO. After all, the wise person always has a backup plan to reach his or her dream, in case the first choice does not come true.

Notes

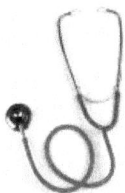

8

Alternatives To A US Doctorate In Medicine or Osteopathic Medicine

Other important alternatives in the health profession to US doctors of medicine or osteopathic medicine.

A.) As you are standing in the hall of life, looking at your future, you have goals to reach and dreams to fulfill. But often this must happen through challenges and adversities. At this stage of the game, you are likely to have committed yourself into working in the health profession. You enjoy being involved in alleviating human sufferings through your service and dedication. Nevertheless, you need preparation, proper skills and knowledge, and a valid license to be fully functional. If graduating as a physician from one of the appropriate schools in Canada or the United States of America does not seem to be feasible for any reasons, remember you have other alternatives.

Your choices include not only the Allopathic Schools (MD), or the osteopathic schools (DO), but also the podiatric school, dental school, optometric school, or veterinary medical school.

1 **A Doctor of podiatric medicine** (DPM) in the USA is a licensed doctor who is an expert that can diagnose and treat conditions pertaining to the foot, ankle and the structures in the leg. In order to qualify, after the four years of college, and after taking the MCAT *(Medical College Admission Test)*, you need to be accepted in a professional doctoral degree that consists of a four-year program followed by two or three years as a resident. After successfully completing the broad certification process, then you are a foot and ankle surgeon certified by the ABPS *(American Board of Podiatric Surgery)*. As a podiatrist, you can also choose solo practice or be associated with other specialists including orthopedist, or join some established private or government sponsored health institutions. For

further details, please consult the AACPM *(American Association of Colleges of Podiatric Medicine)* and other appropriate institutions.

2. What about a career in **Dentistry**. Pursuing a career in oral health care can certainly make a difference in people's life and put a bright and healthy smile on their face. As a dentist you will be able to diagnose, treat and help in preventing diseases of the oral cavity, as well as most of the surrounding areas: hard and soft tissues. In the USA to become a full fledged Dentist, you need four years of undergraduate study with the minimum course prerequisites that include Biology, Chemistry, Biochemistry, English, Physics and Mathematics; other subjects of interests including classes in Humanities, Arts and Social Science; and the official scores from the DAT *(Dental Admission Test)*, as well as letters of recommendation. Then you apply for a doctoral degree either as Doctor of Dental Surgery (DDS) or Doctor of

Dental Medicine (DMD). Some go even further in completing an internship or residency after their degree. There is also a variety of specialties that you can choose from based on your personal interests. For further information, please contact the American Dental Education Association Application Service (CSRAADSAS@ADEA.ORG).

3. As a **Doctor in Optometry**, you belong to the health care team and your role is crucial in people's vision. You get trained to know the structure and function of the eye. You can perform a thorough examination, discover any abnormalities, diagnose and treat the disorders that affect vision or the eye. Prior to your admission into optometry school, you need to finish your undergraduate studies that include the required classes in science and health. Upon admission, you spend four years with the emphasis on acquiring knowledge, and experience in the profession's specific goal. Subsequently, you receive your degree as doctor of optometry (OD)

with the option for further training in subspecialties.

All in all, there is a wide array of options for everyone who wants to pursue a career in the health field at different levels.

4. If you have a genuine love and concern for animals and their well-being, Veterinary Medicine would be a favorable path. In the United States, to become a veterinarian, you need a veterinary degree such as **Doctor of Veterinary Medicine** (DVM) and to be licensed. Preveterinary education is paramount. You will need a B.S, or B.A. degree with required science courses, or at least 60 semester hours in a respectable educational institution. Some Veterinary schools may not require certain official tests, but most of them want your score from *Graduate Record Examination* (GRE), or *Medical College Admission Test* (MCAT). Veterinary School admission is also competitive and the veterinary curriculum is rigorous. The key is to strive for great performance in undergraduate education

with a competitive scientific background and an impressive grade point average that will distinguish you from the pool of qualified applicants.

The Veterinary Medical Schools are accredited by the American Medical Association Council on Education. Once accepted in one of them, you spend four years acquiring the necessary knowledge to become a well rounded expert for a much needed service, covering a wide range of species. For further information, please consult the appropriate authorities, including, WWW.AAVMC. ORG, AVMA.ORG/CAREFORANIMALS, etc.

B.) Should foreign medical schools be an option? If so when and where?

Everyone's situation is unique. Every decision is personal. There cannot be a one-size-fits-all answer to that question. Allow me to state unequivocally, if you live here in the US and intend to stay and practice here, you should do everything that is possible under the sun for admission to an allopathic or osteopathic medical school in the United States before opting for somewhere else. It remains your personal decision. There are many different plausible scenarios, such as the following.

Scenario #1:

You grew up in the United States of America; you went to high school and college here. You apply to US medical schools; unfortunately you are not accepted the first time. Everybody is giving you advice. What do you do? You are still young; you are fresh out of college; you have family and parental support. You should review your credentials and engage in more medically related positions and activities, performing health related community service, volunteering in some medical schools or hospitals, doing some research in the health field, even furthering some graduate studies.

Get acquainted with some known and influential department chairs who can write excellent recommendation letters on your behalf, or take some appropriate post graduate classes, then reposition yourself for the following year with more determination, self confidence, and an improved attitude.

You may also apply to more schools, including a few new ones and consider D.O. schools. You have heard this adage over and over: If at first you don't succeed, try and try again. However, if one year, two years, or more go by and nothing happens, it is prudent to consider other options

Scenario # 2

You have immigrated into the US as an adolescent; you finish high school and college here. You apply to medical schools with transcripts that have equivalent courses here but some were already obtained outside of the US. This means you are still in the process of learning how to fit into the educational systems in the USA; your scores are not high enough to compete but you have the burning desire to be a physician. You may be more easily convinced to look for other options.

Scenario #3

You already went to medical school in a foreign country, and you want to get into the US system and function as a licensed physician in the United States.

There are even a few instances where people go offshore because of financial situations. Whatever the case or the reason may be, you need to make an educated decision. The choice to study medicine abroad and come back to practice as a licensed physician in the US has a lot of ramifications and cannot be taken lightly. Although there are United States citizens and residents who go primarily to the Caribbean, Mexico, Philippines, England, Israel, Ireland, and other countries to study medicine, there are no official statistics to tell us whether or not all of them get what they wanted either in the foreign land or when they came back into the US system. You need to be well informed as to all the steps to be taken before you can become eligible to get into a residency program in the U.S., and avoid disappointment. You must take into consideration the various aspects of any foreign school.

1. Legitimacy and reputation, its standings with the World Health Organization, and access to external organizations' reviews of the schools and qualification of its students to take USMLE exams.

2. Faculty's composition and academic credetials; curriculum's compatibility and parity with US schools, possibility of transfers into US medical schools, as well as its recognition by the United States Department of Education.

3. The rigor of its requirements for admission, and the seriousness of the medical programs not only in basic science but also in clinical—the overall program outline and its standings in the world. Availability of school catalog and website.

4. What are the condition and availability of clinical teaching facilities? What do you know about the possibilities for clinical rotations? Can its

students be accepted for training in some medical centers and affiliated hospitals in the US? You need to be aware that some states forbid foreign students to have clinical rotations in their hospitals.

5. Percentage of students who passed the *United States Medical Licensing Examination* (USMLE) steps 1 and 2 and got into a US residency in the past.

6. Its facilities, labs, libraries, internet, email access and resources, equipment availability, training sites and performance.

7. Stability and security of the host countries, level of freedom and respect regarding religion, socioeconomic living standard, politics, and culture.

8. The cost for the length of stay, as well as the impact of being away from parents, families and friends; availability of financial aid, and the possibility for such a school to meet the US Department of Education's standards for US student loans.

9. The length of the program, the student support program, the dropout rates, and reasons given for such rates.

10. The possibility of not being able to get admitted in the very prestigious residency programs, or very competitive specialties such as neurosurgery, orthopedic surgery, urology...in the United States and often having to settle for a second choice.

As much as possible, you and someone with experience—perhaps your parents—should go there to visit and see what you are getting yourself into. Talk to graduates and current students there. This helps to lower your chances for disappointment. You can also find out whether or not it is a place to stay and practice if things do not work out in the USA; your ability to communicate well and understand the language(s), you should verify all the claims made about that school through independent sources.

HOW CAN A FOREIGN GRADUATE MAKE IT IN THE US SYSTEM?

1. Pass USMLE steps I and II, aiming at being among those who obtain the highest scores. Bear in mind, you are competing with the US graduates. You need to prove that you can do as well as they, if not better. During my fellowship years, I had the distinguished honor of helping as an assistant program director in a residency program. For each foreign candidate, I could not resist asking myself: why is he or she a foreign graduate? What can he offer that a US graduate cannot? How well can he function in our system? Will he be available and fully committed here or elsewhere? What is the immigration status? Based on the answers we could come up with, that would help us make a decision one way or the other. Your scores definitely matter when being considered for residency.

2. Tend to your application, the length, and content of your letter, the way the whole package looks. How would

you feel looking at an application with coffee stain, a barely visible picture, or a hardly readable note? Who has time to give extra effort to understand one candidate's application when there are hundreds more ready to go?

3. Be in step with technology where it is applicable: email address, emailing, being able to visit websites to answer most of your questions. Beware of the background noise when an authorized person from a program calls.

4. Be prepared to live with the label of foreign or offshore graduate vs. a US graduate. It should not bother you, since this is a fact. The key is to remain committed to being a caring, skilled, and compassionate physician.

5. For further information, please go directly to the appropriate sources; consult the organizations that can provide much more detail, including the National Association of Advisors for the Health Professions (NAAHP), the American Association of International Medical Graduates

(AAIMG): WWW.AAIMG.COM/CRITERIA/INDEX. HTML, The Complete Guide to Foreign Medical Schools in Plain English by Nilanjan Sen, and many more. There you can find all that is mentioned above and much more.

C.) Please remember there are still other alternatives in taking care of sick people. A very popular and promising approach is held by chiropractors who use natural technique to work in human heath and disease process. In fact through manual and conservative treatments, the **Chiropractic Doctor** seeks to address neurological, skeletal or soft tissue complaints. For further information, please feel free to consult with the American Chiropractic Association, WWW. AMERCHIRO.ORG.

Notes

Part 2:

Secrets To Becoming A
Great Resident, Then Physician

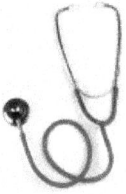

9
The Residency Program

Do you remember what you went through to find a medical school to study medicine? Well, here comes another hurdle to overcome. After four years in medical school, because all has gone more or less as expected, you have managed to meet all the requirements, to pass all the courses. Now you have to choose a residency program. This is usually less painful. Generally, after graduating from an accredited US medical school, you should be able to get to a residency program. You may not necessarily get where and what you want, especially if you go for the very competitive programs in urology, dermatology, otolaryngology, orthopedic surgery, or neurosurgery, for example. But overall you should get a decent residency acceptance.

During the fourth year there are, again, some major decisions to be taken: are you going to be an internist or a family practitioner, or are you going to choose to be a specialist? You must submit your list of programs from different hospitals for considerations on time.

Then come the magic words: **match day**. This is a special time in March where fourth year medical students throughout the United States will find out where they are going to do their residency. This also depends on your area of interest, based on your personality, dreams, and basic pursuits in life. Before you know it, the four years are over, you are graduated, and you are matched to your chosen specialty and medical institution.

Again, what leads you to decide on a type of practice? Your choice should not be made solely on the basis of how much money you can make. Always select what you like, what you are comfortable doing, and what can help others.

Revisit the initial reasons why you got into medicine. You are embarking on a lifetime commitment, day-in and day-out, 24/7, week after week, month after month, and year after year. You need a field that provides a good balance between your personal dreams and your career. So, based on the opportunities offered, your type of personality, your character, your lifestyle, the length of residency for the specialty, the requirements to be board certified in a given specialty, and its income, you can opt for one of the multiple specialties such as obstetrics and gynecology, neurosurgery, neurology, internal medicine, family practice, hospitalist, anesthesiology, radiology, general surgery, orthopedics, psychiatry, dermatology, pediatrics, and many others, as well as subspecialties.

Again, please remember that some fields are more competitive and more demanding than others and may require many more years of residency. Some programs are even pyramidal, meaning the number of residents shrinks as they move up from year to year. For example, a program in neurosurgery may start with twelve residents the first year, but by the time they finish, only two or three may be left. The rest may have to start from scratch in another program.

Do not yield to others' pressures. After all is said and done, you will have to face yourself in the mirror every day. Immediately after you become qualified for any certification, starting with USMLE steps 1 and 2 to your highest specialization, please take the test right away while the materials are fresh in your head, especially if you have not yet committed yourself to full practice. You are still shielded from a lot of daily exigencies of life. Do not put it off. The average residency program is three years, but some specialties may require a transitional year. You may even go for a fellowship. The bottom line is you are advancing in your career. You are now getting paid to learn and be trained. Do not put off the exams you are qualified to take. Do not blow it with extravagance.

You have heard all kinds of tales about residency. The truth is things have improved considerably, and more steps are to be taken to make it more appropriate. Now you are dealing with real patients who are usually very nice. They look up to you to help them get well. Their well-being is paramount. All you need to do is to be responsible and respectful, to look nice and clean. Answer the questions, you can, candidly. Those you cannot answer, you say you do not know and you will follow through and get back to them. Do not play God; know your limits; do not give out false information. Do not make promises you cannot keep. Remember, a good medical student usually makes a good resident. A good resident usually makes a good attending physician.

RESIDENCY 101

Here are ten steps to becoming an outstanding resident:

1. Cultivate a proactive, positive attitude and capitalize on your potentialities. Never miss a moment to increase your knowledge and better yourself as a whole.

2. Work smart, efficiently, and thoroughly; and remain prudent. Be available. When you are called or paged, answer promptly and intelligently to questions asked. By the same token, when all your work

is done, be reachable, but go to the library or to your study hall or room.

If you are always present in the unit, your work will never be over. The staff will call you for everything in the wee hours of the night because you are there. They may even list your name as the resident notified if something happens, even though you are not on call. A staff member, the nurse, will contact any resident available, especially after regular hours. The hospitals documents when Dr. John Doe was informed of any emergency that may occur; whether you were on call or not. Your name will be written in that incident, that emergency report, even though you were not on call.

Again, be thorough, and be reachable when needed. However, do not be everpresent when not on call, or you will wind up doing the call yourself; especially when something goes wrong or if the resident on call is not that reliable.

3. Begin your day early and finish it late whenever it is required of you.

4. Be pleasant, friendly, courteous, and helpful to everyone, including the nursing staff; try to get along with everybody. Never be the source of a stressful situation.

5. Remain humble and tactful. Do not look for shortcuts. Always ask the attending physician about how he or she wants to manage each patient, what to order, who to consult. Remember, it's the attending's patient. He or She is the one who is fully responsible for the patient's care.

6. Say no evil, and do not be part of any evil doing.

7. Know everything that you can possibly know about your patients before rounds and do not be late and unprepared. You will be surprised at how much you can learn from patients just by spending some time with them, getting their full stories and putting the puzzle together.

Finish your work; do not assign your unfinished task to the colleague on call, unless it is an emergency. Remember, emergencies do not happen every week or every day. For example, do not draw labs at the last minute and then sign them out to the poor soul on call who has a lot to cover plus new admissions and potential codes.

8. Be genuine. Do not try to bluff your way around. Make no waves. The attending physicians have been around. You will be discovered for who you are. Word will get around fast, and there goes your reputation.

9. Do not complain: People may take you for a lazy, grumpy bum. Keep your serenity, even under trials and undeserved humiliation.

10. Try to write legibly, date, and time your progress note, and use your stamp with your beeper or cell number when signing your note.

Notes

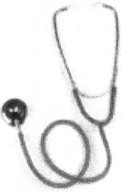

10

How to Be a Great Physician

Nuts and Bolts of
The Practice of Medicine

Bravo! Bravo! Bravo! You have made it. You went to medical school, you finished your residency, and you are board certified. Maybe you are even board certified in a subspecialty. This is great and beyond belief.

Guess what? Now real life begins! You need to have a life: get married if you want to; have children if you so desire; pay your bills as you must; earn a decent living; and enjoy some well deserved benefits, while taking care of all the patients who need your help. It is an innate desire for all normal people to be the best in whatever they do. You are no exception.

As a physician you need knowledge, experience, and wisdom; but above all, you need the proper attitude and good common sense as you try to orient yourself in the rewarding yet challenging field of medicine. Do you know what you want? What do you do? Do you become a full time appointee in a prestigious teaching hospital? Or do you open an office? Do you do both or neither?

Becoming a full-time faculty hospital employee may be appropriate for some. Others may want to open an office and stay on their own. There is no specifically wrong or right way to go. However, you should always ask people who have been around; get feedback from a few people you trust before diving in.

When you start, unless you have a lot of money, or you have inherited a practice from your mom or dad, you should diligently manage your finances. Opening an office is a thrill, but it can be very expensive also, especially in the beginning. You may need to take a loan to rent a decent place, buy or lease equipment, advertise, for marketing, for employees, and so forth. These expenses are going to take a big part of the money that is not yours, plus you need to pay yourself. Before you know it, all the loans start to become due, including your student loans. You can barely pay the minimum. You feel trapped and overwhelmed. Patients are trickling in slowly, the insurance companies are paying you peanuts after hundreds of denials, and family members are questioning your judgment, while everybody else who sees you as a doctor knows that you are rich and you do not dare to tell them otherwise.

If you choose to work in the hospitals, you are new, you may be stuck with the most difficult patients with little or no insurance, and you have bad on call schedules. Some patients with state insurance may believe it is an entitlement; some may give you a hard time. You are on call almost every weekend, and every other day. Your student loans are due. You wake up depressed, frustrated, and wondering why you went through so much trouble. Here is some advice to decrease your level of frustration and your anxiety:

1. If possible, get a part-time or even a full-time job at a hospital, preferably a teaching institution, so you can have

some money coming in and remain intellectually challenged, if only at the beginning.

2. Refrain from starting any big expenses that you know or have heard of or seen doctors do. You will have time for that but not now. You need to breathe and live. The time for showing off is not at this moment, if ever!

3. Take some of the salary you are earning from your hospital employment and get yourself incorporated as a professional corporation, either under your name or another name you like (not your inlaws, please!), with a tax identification number (TIN).

4. Find a practice with a decently busy office, preferably in a different specialty so you won't compete but complement each other. Rent some space from it for a couple of hours, and then days, per month, for a flat fee with everything covered (rent, utilities, phone, and secretary).

5. Apply to most of the insurance panels available.

6. Get your professional liability insurance. It is expensive, so make sure it is worth it. Find out if you are covered while you are on the hospital premises and for what procedures.

7. Then start seeing some patients in coordination with your schedule on your main job.

8. Have a diligent, honest biller who knows what he or she is doing.

9. Beware of so-called friends who will contact you for all kinds of rosy adventures. Like they say, if it is too good to be true, believe it is too good to be true and stay away. Be careful of your hard-earned license, because ignorance of the principles is not an excuse in a court of law.

10. Be patient. Patience is a rare virtue but very important in the field of medicine. If you are competent, caring, and courteous, without shame,

arrogance, strife, and villainy, time is on your side to become a satisfied and distinguished physician.

Be it in a medical center with affiliated hospitals or in private practice, your goal must remain: be an outstanding physician and do not compromise yourself; do not follow any bad examples.

THE HOSPITAL SETTING

Hospital settings are somewhat different from a private office. The hospital has rules, regulations, red tape, administration, ancillaries, and regular workers who usually do not see things through the eyes of the physicians.

But a hospital has several key advantages:

1. It bestows upon you the prestige of being affiliated with a teaching hospital, where you can further your learning experience.

2. It gives you the elated pleasure of teaching students and residents. By doing so, you are forced to be up to date and engaged in a continuous process of learning.

3. It gives you exposure to patients with challenging conditions, case presentations that can really help you broaden your knowledge and experience.

4. You will be remunerated. It may not be much, but you can budget on it.

5. You can admit your patients for acute or urgent care and procedures that you may not be able to provide in a private office.

So what do you do to navigate through the hospital setting?

1. Network and be a team player.

2. Respect everybody and be friendly to all, with no exceptions.

3. Be careful about the image you project and about your reputation. Once established, be it true or not, it will be hard to shake off.

4. Work with the residents. Do not humiliate them publicly if you can possibly avoid doing so. Remember, you once were one of them. So be

reasonable and understanding, give them clear guidance, and let them know unequivocally what you expect from them in general and how to deal with each of your patients.

5. When you admit a patient, have a clear plan for quick and thorough workup and discharge. Most hospital staff will love you for it.

6. If you are a specialist, acting as consultant, be as prompt in seeing the patients as humanly and medically possible. Do not let the residents do all the work and make all the recommendations without you actually examining the patient yourself. As much as possible, write a clear, legible consult, try to answer the specific question that made them call you as an expert, and give a courtesy call to the referring doctor to discuss the patient. If this is not possible, at least inform the resident assigned to the patient of what you recommend and of any urgent order.

7. Administration is there to run the hospital efficiently and keep it in the black. Try your best to be a team player. Learn about their rules and regulations, and let them know also what you can do and what is not possible from the beginning. Overall, they will work with you. Once in a while, you will find a few individuals who want to run you over and play doctor or treat you like nobody. This is a rare exception. When that happens, follow the chain of command and find a respectable, civil way to make your viewpoint known. Always give people the benefit of doubt. A lot of problems and conflicts arise from lack of understanding, and miscommunications. If, finally, you are convinced that the situation is unbearable, you can choose another setting. This is what is great in medicine; you will find a place where you are able to practice safely and securely.

Private Practice

For a while, I have asked my patients what they expect from a doctor and a medical office. Based on what they say and my personal experience, here are a few insights as to what makes a successful practice.

1. Front desk. You need someone who is well mannered and with a sharp mind, a nice tone of voice, excellent phone manners, and an enthusiastic, positive attitude. This person should be quick thinking and able to care for almost anything that goes on in the office, with a sense of ownership, rather than an indecisive person who has to come to you to ask what color of sticky notes to buy.

2. Waiting room. Keep the waiting room clean, well ventilated, and at a comfortable temperature setting, with appropriate, reasonably current magazines that can be seen by any patient or family member (discarding those that are over two months old).

3. Availability in a timely fashion. All patients want their doctors to be available when they need them. So have a system in place whereby they can reach you or leave a message. Based on the type or urgency of the message; at least have someone return the call. Have regular and known office hours so that the "emergency" cases can be squeezed in right away. Always give the patients a follow-up appointment based on their needs and their condition, tell them to call the emergency number when immediate face-to-face medical attention is required and you are not available right away or the condition cannot be addressed in a private office setting. For example, a patient with sudden onset of the worst headaches in her/his life who then becomes unresponsive must go straight to emergency department by ambulance.

Always encourage patients to call your office for any new development or to inquire about their labs results. This will help in keeping you on your toes for critical lab values. If you give them a new medication, have your office call them in the following twenty-four to forty-eight hours to find out how they are doing.

4. Listening ears, communication. Nowadays, medicine is geared towards volume. This shortens the dialogue between patients and doctors. Nevertheless, the patients want a doctor who can spend some time listening to their complaints and conveying the sense that he or she cares and sympathizes with them and is willing to do his or her best to help them.

Think about preparing and submitting to your regular patients once a year or so a "patient satisfaction survey" to give them the chance to convey their needs, expectations, wishes, and opinions about their relationship with the doctor. In that survey, ask them about access, responsiveness, and professionalism of the office, reasonableness of time in scheduling appointment, how satisfied they are with the office, the staff, the doctors; how convenient it is to come to the office, how likely they are to recommend your service to others, and any additional comments or complaints. Their feedback can help you in many ways.

Be careful about the words you use in front of patients and body language they read when you are seeing them. I still remember when, one late evening after seeing a lot of patients, I told a middle-aged woman, "Your brain MRI shows a small tumor; we need to do a biopsy. There is nothing to worry about; it is superficial. Most likely it is nothing, or a cyst or something benign, but we just want to be one hundred percent sure. So tomorrow I will send you to see the neurosurgeon, Dr. _____. But again don't worry about it." The patient said, "Yes." She seemed to understand everything I said and left my office. I went my way.

By midnight, I got a phone call from the emergency room. The ER doctor told me the patient told him I said she "has a brain tumor that is so bad there is nothing I can do about it. She needs an autopsy of the brain." This is a real story. The patient heard three words:

tumor, nothing, and biopsy. The last word she changed to autopsy.

Luckily, I usually have a staff member with me in those cases. But I hope you realize that you cannot emphasize enough how important it is to be careful not only with what you say—the words you use—but especially what the patients hear and understand. We should make them repeat it and explain it.

Sometimes, we overlook the fact that what is a routine condition for us doctors, day in and day out, is for each patient a once-in-a-lifetime event. A neurologist sees thousands of strokes, but for the patients this is the worst thing that happens to them. Even if they have heard or seen it before with others, they never thought it could ever happen to them. A cardiologist sees countless myocardial infarctions; for the patient this is the first. The patient is frightened. The doctor must remember that and convey some assurance, some hope, without lying.

5. Competency and bedside manner. Patients love to know that their doctor

is knowledgeable and thorough. Be kind to the patients. Be courteous and considerate to them and their family members, regardless of the situation.

Every human being can have a bad day. If on a rare occasion you meet an unreliable or noncompliant patient, keep your cool. "Do no harm" encompasses the emotional and psychological as well as the physical. Do not take the patient's abuse personally. Remain dignified and professional. If absolutely nothing works, excuse yourself, remain silent, and have another doctor attend to the patient. He or she may even complain about you; but you and your conscience will be at peace. Remember, you see thousands of patients who are happy and satisfied, so do not let one or two make you bitter or alter your commitment to help. Remember why you went into medicine. Furthermore, patients and family members may forgive your shortcomings if you treat them with respect, if you listen to them, if you take some time to explain to them what is going on.

6. Treat your office as a business. You may be shocked to read this in a book written by a colleague. But dear friends, it is the truth.

Business should not be a dirty word for doctors. You are in the business of caring for patients. By the same token you must pay rent, utilities, employees, taxes, and insurance; and you must take care of your family and personal needs. You cannot run the office like everybody else does. You need to be unique, even better than the rest, without being a cutthroat, miserable, disgusting drudge.

How do you do that?

1. **Make them feel good.** When the patients come, treat them right. Show them you are more interested in them than in their money or their insurance papers. Let your competent receptionist or manager (if you can afford one) handle the money part. Do not make them wait for hours while joking on the phone.

Make sure your office remembers their birthday, special dates, or events in their lives and acknowledges them by a card or a note. In the follow-up visit, ask them about their spouses and their kids (all information you can get from the initial intake form). They will be impressed if you remember their kids' or grandkids' names. If they mention a sickness in the family, make a note of it and ask your office to call them days or weeks later to inquire how things are. Believe me; the best advertising is by words of mouth from satisfied patients.

2. **Community involvement.** Organize and sponsor events; let the community newspaper know of your existence; have your office do press releases, food drives, toy collections for the needy; offer to write a short article for them every now and then; give them some interviews; help the needy; organize a health fair in correlation with churches and other community centers. Be there when your help is needed and appropriate.

3. **Networking.** Keep a list of email and street addresses of all the patients and potential patients in the

community. Have a four to six page brochure and mail it or have it delivered to them. As a specialist, send a report to the colleague who refers the patient to you and ask the patient to return to his or her PMD for follow-up.

4. **Patient education.** Your office TV should be providing useful information for your patients' health instead of all kinds of popular shows that tend to be stressful and may not help to keep your patient physically and emotionally healthy.

5. **Time management.** All of us have the same twenty-four hours in each day; the difference is in how we use them. For example, I see doctors' signs or hear them tell their patients on the phone, "Our office hours are Monday to Friday from 9 A.M. to 7 P.M., Saturday from 8 A.M. to 5 P.M." When most patients hear that or read such a sign, a lot will show up only on Saturdays, or else early morning or in the evening. They will stop by nonchalantly at their convenience.

What about the doctor's convenience and the office staff's convenience?

The efficient approach is to have some early morning hours on certain days and some evening hours on different days, making sure everybody has an appointment. Give them two options, morning or evening, but not a fifty-hour window. When you pack your office by block of patients, then you can dedicate some time for chart reviews, lab reviews, note completion, becoming better organized and more time efficient. And your family will appreciate it. But the fifty-hour window will force you to bring work home. So you will never have time for self and family. Try it, and you will be surprised. Most patients will comply, and you will get much more accomplished daily.

6. **Hospital visits to see patients.** Try early mornings or late evenings. During the day, you have a full staff talking and intermingling. Sometimes your chart is in the hands of the social worker, the resident or the nurse. You sit to write, everybody is talking, you cannot concentrate, and your

patients are not even there. They went for a test. You waste time that way. When you are on call, especially on weekends, whenever possible, dedicate some specific hours in the morning or evening to see all the patients.

7. **Phone calls.** Train your office to ask all callers whether or not it is an emergency. That way you can block out a specific time when you are less busy to return calls. Patients hate it when doctors answer calls while they are being examined. Of course every situation has its particularities. But it is worth finding ways to maximize the use of one's time. The only time we have is the present moment. Why waste it?

8. **Financial security.** It is unanimous: doctors work a lot. But how much do they have financially to show for all the hours they put in? The scary part is that many doctors do not even know how much money they earn except when, at the end of the year, their accountants tell them.

This has got to stop! You should have a budget. Stop being sentimental, emotionally attached to offices and activities that do not help you financially. Why have three offices, with one supporting the other two? Reevaluate. Share or close those that are ruining you. Every medical office should be able to support itself. Otherwise, you must reevaluate and act. Do you have a budget? Do you have an investment portfolio? Do you have a will? Do you have asset protection? Every doctor should have a financial advisor (besides an accountant), a personal physician, and a lawyer. The time to do it is now, not later, not next week or next month. Pick up the phone now and get your finances in order.

9. **Family life.** Ask the spouses of doctors, most of them will be up in arms because docs have no time for them. Ask the children; they will echo the spouses' cries.

Doctors are always on the run. Many of them have the false sense of being the center of the world; if they are gone, their thinking goes the world will come to an abrupt standstill. Beloved, it is time to realize "there is a time for every purpose under heaven." Please, dedicate some quality time to your partner, your children, your loved ones.

After all is said and done, when you put down the gloves and hang up the coat, the only ones left by your side are your loved ones. Be careful they are not eaten up with resentment and regret. So be a great physician, but do not exclude your family. Squeeze them in, the same way you squeeze in someone else who needs medical care. Yours want some tender loving care.

And for your family's sake, visit your personal doctor regularly and be compliant.

10. **Ethical behavior.** Be ethical and avoid greed. As you are gaining more exposure, you need to stay humble and be careful. All kinds of people want to see you and be seen or associated with you. Have an initial no for everyone, especially those you do not know.

They will come with all kinds of proposals for tests for patients; they will show all kinds of great charts where other offices make a lot of money using this and that. The golden rule: if you did not learn it from all your training, if it is not recommended by prestigious, respectable medical or scientific journals or medical associations, if you do not see the diagnostic or treatment benefits for your patients, send them away. Beware! Investigate thoroughly any companies that want you to work for them or with them. Know what is legally and ethically acceptable early in your career.

Do not see patients or order test for patients or perform tests for patients who have no symptoms, no findings. By the same token, do not be insensitive to the genuine patient who is suffering. Some pathology may take time to show signs that can be picked up by the doctor. You must be careful not to insult the patients or ignore their complaints. At times, there is a tiny fine line between what is true and real and what is purely suggestive, but you must walk that line, using your knowledge, training, experience, humility, history, best judgment, enlightened conscience, values, and ethical conviction. If ever you have to err, let it be on the side of a clear conscience, without ignoring the patient's complaints.

The well-being of the patient must remain paramount. In the course of your practice, it is possible to experience some low points, but let it never be because you knowingly and willfully engage in something unethical. I tease my few physician friends every now and then by telling them that all physicians should be believers. Why? Only God is truly on our side. You may be one hundred percent great for thousands of patients; you may save countless lives; and then you have one bad moment; you make one mistake. The patient, the patient's family, the press, the state, the insurer, those who envy you just for being a physician—all of them will have a field day. If it turns out it was a false accusation, when you are vindicated, almost no one will hear about that part. This is a strange situation where you are guilty until you are found innocent. So be careful! Stay the course!

Remember your calling and respect the Hippocratic Oath:

"I do solemnly swear, by whatever I hold most sacred, that I will be loyal to the profession of medicine and just and generous to its members.

"That I will lead my life and practice my Art in uprightness and honor.

"That into whatsoever home I shall enter it shall be for the good of the sick and the well of the utmost of my power and that I will hold myself aloof from wrong and from corruption and from the tempting of others to vice.

"That I will exercise my Art, solely for the cure of my patients and the prevention of disease and will give no drugs and perform no operation for a criminal purpose and far less suggest such a thing.

"That whatsoever I shall see or hear of the lives of men and women which is not fitting to be spoke, I will keep inviolably secret.

"These things I do promise and in proportion as I am faithful to this oath, may happiness and good repute be ever mine, the opposite if I shall be foresworn."

OVERALL, THE AUTHENTIC PHYSICIAN SHOULD SHOW:

Magnanimity — natural care and concern for others, with noble sentiment

Education — commitment to be knowledgeable, efficient, and experienced

Dedication — to the causes pertaining to patients and health care

Integrity of character

Compassion — love, respect, tolerant and responsible, humble and simple

Availability, accountability, altruism

Loyalty

Discipline in personal life, dynamism, determination

Organizational skills

Communication skills — common sense to deal with patients, family, and others

Trustworthiness and **truthfulness** — with honesty, integrity, and ethics

Optimism — with objectivity

Reliability and **resiliency**

Notes

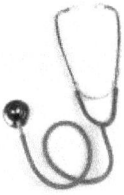

11
Doctors Are People, Too!

A book that only presents a rosy, wonderful, glamorous picture of doctors would be somehow incomplete. The public and aspiring doctors should also know that other side in the life of those who take care of patients. The Bible says, in Luke 12:48, "...For unto whomsoever much is given, of him shall be much required..." It is an undeniable fact that a doctor has received—or, better yet, acquired—a lot of knowledge. The practice of medicine requires a lifetime commitment to constant learning for the specific objective of serving others, taking care of the sick, including the underserved, to alleviate their suffering.

We do it tirelessly, with total dedication, sometimes under dire circumstances, with long hours and difficult conditions. However, no matter how strange this may sound, doctors are human beings. Some seem to forget or ignore that fact. As proof, consider the following scenario: A patient comes to see the doctor. He complains of neck pain radiating to the upper extremities, some cramps, numbness, and tingling on and off. The examination is normal. What do you do?

1. You say, "Well, the examination is normal; here are some Motrin and muscle relaxants; use them as needed." After explaining how to take the medications, what to look for as side effects and allergic reactions, and what to do in such a case, you shake the patient's hand and say, "take care of yourself and I'll see you in a week." But there is always a chance the patient may not come back. You may miss a herniated disc that is pressing on the nerves, an early abscess, an infarct, or even a mass causing further damage. The patient continues with the discomfort, using the Motrin and the muscle relaxants. Three months, six months later, he goes to see another doctor. This time, tests are done with significant

positive findings. The patient may decide to sue you, the first doctor, for failing to address the issue on time. The case may be dismissed further down the line. But when the doctor's insurer asks him annually, "Have you ever been sued?" guess what the right answer should be? Guess how the insurance carrier will view this?

2. On the other hand, if you decide to be careful and to rule out the possibility of missing some pathological finding, here are some possible scenarios: you order a cervical spine MRI for possible disc herniation or/and may do or refer for a nerve conduction study and electromyography to rule out or document neuroradiculopathy.

Depending on the type of insurance the patient has, you or someone from your office may need to invest the time to call, be put on hold, and wait until, after answering questions and giving reasons for the test, you get an authorization. If the insurer is not satisfied or not convinced of the necessity for the test, the person at the other end may tell you that a doctor-to-doctor conference is needed or a form will be mailed or faxed to the office to explain necessity and then will be considered for approval.

When the approval is given, it is sent with the note that approval does not guarantee payment. If it is an insurer that does not require prior approval, the test can be done but payment denied because the insurer can hire another licensed physician to say the test was unnecessary. Even after payment, the insurance company can go back—after you use the money for operating expenses and salaries—and declare the test was not necessary and the values were not reliable and the insurer wants its money back. In the worst case, the patient may not even remember that the tests were performed one or two years ago. Then the insurer wants to investigate.

A dentist, an orthopedist, a gynecologist, an internist—any health care provider—may have a payment denied or return payment required afterward. Cornered from all directions, the doctor may need to find a competent lawyer and then find a considerable amount of money as a retainer for the attorney to take the case. When the doctor is cleared of wrongdoing, there is still a cloud over his head. And no one is willing to reimburse the money spent to clear the doctor's name.

Patients want us to be always one hundred percent correct. Family members want us to be always available and to answer all their questions and sometime to each and everyone separately, or they will complain. The hospitals expect all the notes and discharge summaries to be signed on time. The hospital's patient advocates and patient relations department want us to answer every complaint, including "not liking the tone of voice" or "the way the answer was given." The nurses and the unit clerks want all charts in the racks, the insurers want us to call to request their approval for every procedure and some medications, including waiting on hold and giving a full explanation for our requests. They also have the rights to hold or deny payments for any reason, even after the approval is given. Hold it, here is the best part:

they decide for us how much our service is worth after we perform it. Could you imagine asking a plumber to come and fix your leaky faucet and telling him, "You are required by law never to refuse to fix my faucet? So come and do it or I'll report you for refusing to provide care. And after you do it, I will decide whether or not to pay you and how much your service is worth"? How many plumbers would stay in business? How many plumbers' children will go into plumbing school?

How can people wonder why there will be a shortage of physicians around 2015? The patients have their advocates, the insurance companies budget in a staff of lawyers to look after their interest, the local hospitals have their representatives. Who really cares or supports the local community doctor who is not expected to be sick, depressed, and lonely? We hear everybody's complaints, concerns. Sometime, some doctors wonder besides God, whether there is anyone out there to see the doctors as human beings, too? The family is complaining, "You are never here." The patient says, "You do not give me enough time." The patient's family

164

wants to ask more questions. The insurer says you can only spend 'x' minutes for each patient. And the hospitals usually agree with the insurers' view of shorter time for patient encounters: doctors must see 'x' patients per day. You are not allowed any mistakes. You must be one hundred percent flawless all the time.

In all fairness, there are instances where some doctors go out of bounds. We must recognize that the insurance companies are there to make money and watch out for any fraud or any misconduct; the lawyers are there to help them and to make a living themselves. Again, there can be a few black sheep in the family, and they should be dealt with. But not everybody should be a suspect. Do not paint all doctors with the same brush. Because when you reduce us to mere survival, when we feel trapped, cornered everywhere, with people always looking over our shoulders, you are affecting our ability to practice medicine, you are forcing us to reconsider our self denying way of life, or to feel depressed and abandoned. Ultimately, all of us are suffering.

Another burning issue that requires everyone's input is the high cost of medical care. Currently, everyone is up in arms because the cost of medical care is skyrocketing. There is a variety of reasons why delivering medical care is so expensive. They include an aging population using more expensive and more sophisticated equipment to prolong life; unhealthy life style factors such as obesity, poor diet, and sedentary life; demand oriented patients who may request every diagnostic test available, along with costly treatment for their symptoms, because a third party is paying; advanced technology; the cost of prescriptions; expensive new drugs; litigation; and fear of being sued. Some may add the payment to the doctors. The truth is that doctors get a small percentage of the cost of care as salary.

It is an undeniable fact that the U.S. is the leader in the medical field. United States health care provides high standards of care. We have an impressive number of Nobel Prize winners in science. But there is definitely an urgent need to get a handle on health care costs.

Anytime you have a profit oriented, capitalistic system, along with partisan politics and personal bias, you are bound to see greed and selfishness. The corporate costs, administrative costs, regulations, and politics all form a distasteful cocktail. Profit oriented organizations want one thing—to be as profitable as possible. Therefore they want to reduce costs to a bare minimum and increase profits to a maximum. In the process, the victims are the patients. The corporations want to do the least amount of testing possible, provide the cheapest medication, with the minimum level of care. Life expectancy and quality of life should not depend on an individual's economic condition. Although the patients sometime feel helpless against some gigantic firm, they turn on the doctor. They can still sue the physician for not providing what they perceive to be adequate care.

All of us must realize that health care is not a privilege; it is a right and a social, humanistic obligation towards all. It is not an optional commodity to obey capitalistic elastic supply and demand for profit principles. Everyone should be insured, have access to competent care, and at the same time be instructed well enough to know that the insurance policy is not an entitlement. Generally, patients do not go out looking for the cheapest care available. Instead they go where they feel comfortable, under recommendations from other people they trust.

Therefore, politicians and legislators should stop sponsoring regulations tailored to special interests under the guise of ways to improve care. Instead, they should focus on resources of providers and the quality of care, and determine the effective ways and means to deliver it. Insurance should be portable anywhere within the U.S. Malpractice claims, litigation, and frivolous lawsuits should be addressed. There should be guidelines. Gross errors, gross negligence (such as amputating the wrong leg) should be referred to medical review boards, which are appropriate panels for reasonable compensation and appropriate punishment or penalty when needed. For an efficient health care system, we should:

1. Make health care available to all, not as an entitlement but as a necessity with no precondition.

2. Have capitation based on specialty and by time spent, while factoring in the average, possible, necessary, tests per group of patients, years of training, and qualifications of providers. This would reduce the chance for so called unnecessary testing, and fraud.

3. Have universal personal data stored and constantly updated, yet accessible only to responsible, qualified medical personnel. This would reduce duplication of tests that are done within a certain amount of time.

4. Have regulations regarding frivolous law suits. There can be no real health care reform without tort reform. For example, a doctor should not have to be sued for recommending a first line medication, the only one available for a specific condition because— unfortunately —the patient develops a severe, catastrophic allergic reaction to such a medication.

5. Doctors should be working with each other, not competing against each other. They should form regional, community based, neighborhood networks, with a multidisciplinary, multispecialty approach at a prepaid rate and self-regulation with general guidelines.

These steps—and others that can be determined by experts in such a domain—would curb the chance for fraud, reduce the incentive for unnecessary tests, and diminish the fear of lawsuits. The idea of having lay people or administrative doctors (who are not actively practicing medicine) decide and regulate on health care is not practical. Only those who are facing the bullets on the battleground, daily in their private offices or in hospitals, know the dilemma they face and can formulate approaches to handle such crises. They should at least be heard.

What medicine needs now is not necessarily more rules and regulations but a revision of those that are already on the books and a call for fairness, equal treatment, and equal representation.

There is a difference between health reform and insurance reform.

Too often, people develop the wrong opinion about the doctors. I saw a survey on the Internet; I was saddened to see that physicians were not the most trusted professionals. When I asked a few patients, one of them who has known me for years told me, the public thinks that "you guys are in it for the money." She tried to exclude me, but I was not concerned for myself, *per se*, but rather for the entire career of medicine. I tried my best to hide my displeasure regarding what people think of us physicians. I know decent doctors who are struggling, and little did they know about what the general public thinks of them. I want to say, "Hello! Is there anybody out there to hear the doctors?" The checks and balances in the just and fair system that our country represents include everyone. I understand mistakes have been made, abuses committed, but one cannot go from one end to the other. The pendulum should not swing from one extreme to the other. It is time for reason to prevail and for us to bring the pendulum back to the middle, where it should be with checks and balances. If physicians cannot be truthful, cannot be trusted, we may as well hang up the lab coats, put the stethoscope, the tuning fork, the hammer in the drawer, and go skip stones at the beach or feed the pigeons.

It is time for America to wake up and see what is happening to the medical field as a whole. It is time for physicians to stick to their oath, remember their values, and be committed to a dedicated service of care for all.

In the medical schools, maybe, the Oath of Hippocrates should be recited in the classroom daily, ethics classes should be mandatory and early in the curriculum, with regular sessions explaining what being a physician should mean in terms of ethics, values, and etiquette.

As usual, when a problem is posed, there are many causes. It is time for a moratorium, a round table about medicine. We need greater involvement, stronger public advocacy, and recognition for what we have been doing. We need better cooperation and harmony among all doctors, all specialties,including MDs, DOs, and the public. After all, doctors are people too!

Regardless of what happens, we must stay the course and be faithful to our post. Keep the faith. Keep hope alive. Do our utmost to make a difference in people's lives. Be true to our callings like the compass is to the pole. We must not be bitter. Let us keep the positive attitude, our heads straight, facing the future, whatever may come our way. We must always remember why we embrace medicine: total commitment to serving the health care needs of all patients.

In case there is anybody who is wondering what the doctors want, how about appreciation and some understanding! We work countless hours daily, often intervening at the late hours of the night, with no time for family, postponing or canceling vacations, dedicating our entire lives to the profession. Of course, it is our choice! But we only hear people's complaints. When everything is fine, it is just silence. Appreciation, self-esteem, and a sense of accomplishment are worth more than money. Psychologists agree human beings need a token of appreciation daily. It builds up your self-esteem and motivates you to do even more. So, let everybody remember: doctors are human beings, too!!!

Notes

Postscript

Being involved in the health system is a rare and distinguished privilege. Being a physician is an awesome opportunity to cause positive change. Practicing modern medicine makes you part of a team that can contribute to the advancement of the frontiers of medicine. If the medical career is woven of many highs and a few lows, overall, this is one of the most rewarding and satisfying endeavors one can embrace; if you have received the sacerdotal call to apply skill and knowledge and provide exemplary, high quality, compassionate care to people in need, please stay the course!

I hope this book has played a positive role in helping you to choose or pursue a career in medicine. I hope it opens a window to the doctor's life.

About the Author

Jean Daniel François graduated from St. Francis College in Brooklyn, New York, in 1980, with a BS in management. He obtained his master's in economics in 1984 from Long Island University (Brooklyn campus). He worked in accounting and finance for a Fortune 500 company until 1986. Then, responding finally to the call of medicine, he went to New York Medical College, in Valhalla, New York, where he obtained his doctorate in medicine in 1992. While doing his residency in neurology at SUNY-Brooklyn Center, he remained involved in his community. He was honored by the American Medical Association for outstanding community service in December 1997. Such an honor was bestowed upon only forty resident physicians from around the United States. Dr. François was privileged to be recognized, along with thirty-nine other doctors who displayed "leadership and a strong commitment to the health of their patients and the community as a whole through community service outreach." During his fellowship in clinical neurophysiology, he served as Assistant Residency Program Director at SUNY-Brooklyn Center. In an effort to broaden his skills to meet the needs of his community, he also obtained a bachelor's degree in theology.

He is currently a practicing neurologist in his private office. He is in charge of the outpatient neurology clinic and Parkinson's disease clinic at a teaching hospital. He is the spiritual leader of a community-based church and the author of many books, a motivational speaker, and a lecturer on topics such as family life, health, spirituality, domestic violence, successful living, and personal finance. Throughout his speeches and presentations, the focus has always been a total commitment to empower everyone to take control of their existence and step out on the road to a fulfilled life.

Dr. François is married to a registered nurse, born as Jocelyne Cole. They have one son, Jean Daniel Jr., and one daughter, Sarah Jocelyne.

Selected Resources

Becker, Christian, Medical School Admission Guide. Minneapolis: Mill City Press, Inc., 2007

Medical School Admission Requirements from the Association of American Medical Colleges

WWW.STUDENTDOCTOR.NET

WWW.AAMC.ORG

WWW.AACOM.ORG

WWW.OSTEOPATHIC.ORG

WWW.AAIMG.COM

WWW.ASPIRINGDOCS.ORG

WWW.FUTUREDOCTOR.NET

WWW.PREMED101.COM

Afterword

"I read your book...and it was GREAT.

I really liked it. I felt like it was right down to earth and made the reader feel very comfortable with the information and made one feel like anyone could do this...It takes you from beginning to end...tackling admission to starting your own practice, which is rare to find in one book. Usually this is found in a series..."

~ Miss Lorraine Alexis

"Dr. François's Book is an eye-opener that is very useful to anyone interested in medicine at any level."

~ Dr. Jean-Etienne Thibaud, MD, DO

"It is amazing how limitless our potential can be. But to figure out which one direction to pursue to realize that potential, one can spend a whole lifetime and still end up clueless.

For the young and impressionable, those who may have one fiber in their body saying 'I can be a doctor'... pick up this book. It will paint the right picture.

It may not be only the glamorous profession as you see on TV, certainly not as effortless as Dr. House makes it appear to be. It will show you which small steps to take in building a solid undergraduate foundation.

For those already in med school or in training … it will make you appreciate fulfillment in small victories. You may realize how blessed you are for making it this far and inspire you further to push your limits.

For those already in practice… reading through this book flies you back in the journey of your life. Sooner or later, as one gets lost in the middle of the long hours, the threat of litigation, the seemingly endless health care system bureaucracy, and the most dangerous distraction… the lure of more and more money, reading this book will remind you of the very reason why you are in this field in the first place. Whether it be is for the science, or by virtue of altruism, this book shall ground you"

~ Dr. Jeaniesar Caluag

Quick Order Form

Email orders: **Jfranc6704@aol.com**

Fax orders to: **718-531-2329**

Call for order at: **718-531-6100**
Have your credit card ready.

Mail in orders at:
    Jean D. François, MD
    P.O. Box 360543
    Brooklyn NY 11236

Please send the following Books, CD, reports:
    I am interested in:

    ☐ Speaking/ seminars/conferences

    ☐ Consulting

    ☐ Other services needed: _____

Name: _____

Address: _____

City: _____State: _____Zip:_____

Telephone: _____

Cell #:_____

Email address:_____

Shipping and handling:
    U.S: $5.00 for first book, $2.00 for each additional.

www.ingramcontent.com/pod-product-compliance
Lightning Source LLC
Chambersburg PA
CBHW051041030426
42339CB00006B/143